如何践行群医学

How to Practise Population Medicine

【英】缪尔·格雷 著
Muir Gray

主　译　王　辰　杨维中
主　审　张孔来
副主审　郭　岩　陈思邈

中国协和医科大学出版社

北　京

Kindle ISBN 978-1-904202-08-0

© Offox Press，2014年

本书原版权所有者为Offox Press（2014年）。未经版权所有者的事先书面许可，不得以任何形式或任何方式将本出版物的任何部分复制或存储在检索系统中。

著作权合同登记号：图字01-2022-0872号

图书在版编目（CIP）数据

如何践行群医学 /（英）缪尔·格雷（Muir Gray）著；王辰，杨维中译. —北京：中国协和医科大学出版社，2022.7

ISBN 978-7-5679-1913-6

Ⅰ.①如…　Ⅱ.①缪…②王…③杨…　Ⅲ.①卫生管理学　Ⅳ.①R19

中国版本图书馆CIP数据核字（2022）第017859号

如何践行群医学

主　　译：王　辰　杨维中
责任编辑：李元君　张　凌　雷　南
封面设计：许晓晨
责任校对：张　麓
责任印制：张　岱

出版发行　**中国协和医科大学出版社**
　　　　　（北京市东城区东单三条9号　邮编100730　电话010-65260431）
网　　址　www.pumcp.com
经　　销　新华书店总店北京发行所
印　　刷　北京联兴盛业印刷股份有限公司
开　　本　787mm×1092mm　　1/16
印　　张　21.5
字　　数　310千字
版　　次　2022年7月第1版
印　　次　2022年7月第1次印刷
定　　价　108.00元
ISBN 978-7-5679-1913-6

翻译团队

主　译

王　辰　中国医学科学院北京协和医学院

杨维中　中国医学科学院北京协和医学院群医学及公共卫生学院

主　审

张孔来　中国医学科学院北京协和医学院基础医学研究所

副主审

郭　岩　北京大学公共卫生学院

陈思邈　德国海德堡大学全球健康研究所

中文版审校专家（按姓氏拼音为序）

毕振强　山东省疾病预防控制中心

单广良　中国医学科学院北京协和医学院基础医学研究所

翟晓梅　中国医学科学院北京协和医学院群医学及公共卫生学院

冯录召　中国医学科学院北京协和医学院群医学及公共卫生学院

赖圣杰　南安普顿大学地理与环境系

乔友林　中国医学科学院北京协和医学院群医学及公共卫生学院

邵瑞太　中国医学科学院北京协和医学院群医学及公共卫生学院

张　敏　中国医学科学院北京协和医学院群医学及公共卫生学院

赵方辉　中国医学科学院肿瘤医院

译　者（按姓氏拼音为序）

陈秋兰　中国疾病预防控制中心

宫恩莹　中国医学科学院北京协和医学院群医学及公共卫生学院

黄蕾如　中国医学科学院北京协和医学院群医学及公共卫生学院

贾萌萌　中国医学科学院北京协和医学院群医学及公共卫生学院

姜明月　中国医学科学院北京协和医学院群医学及公共卫生学院

冷志伟　中国医学科学院北京协和医学院群医学及公共卫生学院

李晋磊　中国医学科学院北京协和医学院群医学及公共卫生学院

马礼兵　桂林医学院附属医院

马雪迪　中国医学科学院北京协和医学院群医学及公共卫生学院

亓蔚然　中国医学科学院北京协和医学院群医学及公共卫生学院

钱　捷　中国医学科学院北京协和医学院群医学及公共卫生学院

曲翌敏　中国医学科学院北京协和医学院群医学及公共卫生学院

苏琪茹　深圳儿童医院

苏小游　中国医学科学院北京协和医学院群医学及公共卫生学院

孙艳侠　中国医学科学院北京协和医学院群医学及公共卫生学院

佟训靓　北京医院

王　晴　中国医学科学院北京协和医学院群医学及公共卫生学院

王　也　中国医学科学院北京协和医学院群医学及公共卫生学院

徐韵韶　中国医学科学院北京协和医学院群医学及公共卫生学院

杨　娇　中国医学科学院北京协和医学院群医学及公共卫生学院

杨　津　中国医学科学院北京协和医学院群医学及公共卫生学院

伊赫亚　中华预防医学会

张　娟　中国医学科学院北京协和医学院群医学及公共卫生学院

张　婷　中国医学科学院北京协和医学院群医学及公共卫生学院

张惺惺　中国医学科学院北京协和医学院群医学及公共卫生学院

赵　健　中国医学科学院北京协和医学院群医学及公共卫生学院

赵艺皓　中国医学科学院北京协和医学院群医学及公共卫生学院

译 者 的 话

　　《如何践行群医学》（*How to Practise Population Medicine*）是群医学主要倡导者牛津大学缪尔·格雷（Muir Gray）教授的著作。为向读者介绍践行群医学的理念和技能，北京协和医学院群医学团队引进并组织翻译了该著作。2021年，我们团队曾翻译出版了由缪尔·格雷、新西兰学者乔纳森·格雷（Jonathon Gray）和卡瑞娜·麦克哈迪（Karina Mchardy）共同编著的《群医学》（*Population Medicine*），在学界引起了广泛关注，多位读者与我们取得联系，共同探讨群医学的理念与实践，推动了群医学学科发展。《医师报》报社与中国医药卫生文化协会主办了"2021我与好书有个约会·医界好书"活动，《群医学》入选了"管理类十大医学好书"。在此，我们对社会各界给予群医学学科建设与发展的关心和支持致以诚挚的感谢！

　　《如何践行群医学》全书共11章，第一章为群医学——21世纪的新职责，主要从群医学的基本理念出发，论述了临床医生的七大职责；第二至十一章分别从价值最大化、减少资源浪费和提高可持续性、减少不公平、促进健康和预防疾病、设计以人群为基础的整合型体系、为供给体系建立工作网络、患者参与、为人群编制预算、知识管理以及创新和保持正确的文化10个方面阐述如何践行群医学。

　　群医学是一门新兴学科，其思想、理念、内涵、理论体系以及对实践的指导都需要不断丰富和发展。自开始建设北京市教委高精尖学科、成立群医学及公共卫生学院等工作以来，协和医学院又举办了6届中外学者参与的群医学及公共卫生论坛，设置了群医学的课程体系并开始授课，这些举措都进一步推动了群医学学理及学术体系的发展。目前协和医学院群医学团队将群医学定义更新为：群医学是运用、融合当代医学及相关学科的知识、技术、艺术和学术，动员现实可及的资源，从健康促进及疾病的预防、诊断、控制、治疗、康复等方面，统筹个体卫生行为与群体卫生行动，促进人际和谐及人与环境友好，推动健康公平，作为公共卫生的医学基础，实现人群整体与长远健康效益最大化的一门医学学科。协和医学院群医学学科建设的举措已经产生了积极的影响。教育部等四部门下发的《关于开展高水平公共卫生学院建设的通知》中，明确提出要加强群医学相关方向研究，以推进公共卫生多学科交叉研究。一些高校已经开设了群医学课程，还有少数高校已建立了群医学系。

本书是由协和医学院群医学团队与北京大学、中国疾病预防控制中心、中华预防医学会、德国海德堡大学、英国南安普顿大学的同仁们共同努力完成翻译的。在反复校对的过程中，我们进一步体会到作者所处的社会环境及卫生体系与我国不尽相同，加之群医学涉及众多学科，部分英文词汇翻译可能难于达意，甚或存在错误。因此，本书的排版继续采用与《群医学》相同的方式，即原文与译文双语对应排版，便于帮助读者对照原文领悟作者本意。欢迎读者继续与我们联系，帮助我们完善翻译。

《如何践行群医学》双语本可作为群医学、临床医学、公共卫生、卫生管理等专业本科生，以及研究生或研修生的教材或教学辅助资料，也可供从事群医学教学实践的专业技术人员和管理人员参考使用。

群医学或是一次中国医学界领衔于世界的重大机遇。北京协和医学院将继续编著群医学系列专著和教材，开设适用于不同人群的课程体系。望有志之士与我们同思、共为、共享，推动群医学学科进一步繁荣。

王　辰　杨维中

于北京东单北极阁三条31号

2021年6月16日

目录 Contents

目录 Contents

Chapter 1
POPULATION MEDICINE — A NEW RESPONSIBILITY FOR THE 21st CENTURY

第一章
群医学——21世纪的新职责

This chapter will:

- focus on resource constraints, particularly the finite resource of clinician time;
- explain why clinicians feel their sole responsibility lies with the patient in front of them, a situation that arose from an era when the patient paid the doctor directly;
- describe how that relationship changes when healthcare is funded by the whole population, including people who have needs the same as those who are being treated but who have not accessed the service because of reasons outwith their control, such as language difficulties.

By the end of the chapter, you will have developed an understanding of:

- the changing responsibility of the clinician, particularly the doctor, in an era in which healthcare is funded by the whole population and not just by the patients who consult doctors;
- the dual responsibility for clinicians who manage services;
- the new responsibility of the clinician to and for the whole population and the actions they need to take to discharge that responsibility.

■ The traditional responsibility of doctors

Since Hippocrates, the traditional responsibility that doctors have felt to the patient in front of them either on the other side of the desk or lying in bed. This responsibility entailed complete loyalty to the individual patient, and a commitment of resources without consideration of cost.

However, in practice, clinicians have become accustomed to limiting the use of one resource to individual patients in order to ensure that is available to all. This finite resource that the clinician limits so that all patients might benefit is time. If a clinician did not limit the time given to one patient, there would be no time for other patients-indeed, clinicians would rarely get home. This practice has gone on for years despite the knowledge that not only many of a clinician's patients want more time but also that some patients would report a better outcome if more time had been invested in their care. It could be argued that clinicians have not rationed their time with sufficient rigour and, as a consequence, have suffered burnout, a problem that will become more common as the pressure on resources for healthcare intensifies.

本章涉及内容：

- 关注资源有限问题，特别是临床医生有限的时间资源；
- 解释临床医生认为自己只需要对诊治的患者负责的原因，这一意识从患者直接向医生付费的时代延续而来；
- 描述当卫生保健（healthcare）的费用来自于全人群提供时，这种关系是如何变化的，包括那些接受治疗的患者和有着同样需要，但是因为语言困难等客观原因而没有获得治疗的人群。

在本章末，读者将会深入理解：

- 临床工作者，尤其是医生责任的变化，特别是在一个医疗保健资源来自全人群提供而不仅仅来自于寻诊患者提供的时代；
- 管理和服务的临床工作者具有双重责任；
- 临床工作者应当对整个人群承担新责任并付诸行动。

■ 传统意义上医生的责任

从希波克拉底时代起，医生就认为他们只需要向自己诊桌旁或病床上的患者负责。这种传统责任要求医生全身心救治每名患者，保证资源充足，无须考虑成本。

然而，在实践中，临床医生们已经习惯尽可能减少在个体患者身上花费的时间，以确保所有患者都能得到诊治。时间资源有限，限制个人时间消耗能让所有患者获益。如果临床医生不限制单个患者的诊疗时间，那么其他患者就将无法获得应有的诊疗时间，而医生自己也无法下班回家。虽然许多患者都希望获得更多的诊疗时间，而且这样会让他们感觉诊疗效果更好，但是限制患者诊疗时间的做法已经持续多年。可以说，不能严格地分配时间不仅让医生精疲力竭，而随着医疗资源紧缺的压力加剧，这个问题还将变得更加普遍。

■ Deriving greater value from resources

Although time is finite, the benefits of face-to-face time can be enhanced, for example, by using online resources to extend the consultation. Although money is also finite, unlike time it cannot be extended in the same way. Money is inelastic: money spent on one patient cannot be spent on another. Thus, if care is to be extended to patients other than those already being seen by a busy service, greater value will need to be derived from existing resources. This represents a new challenge, entailing new responsibilities for clinicians.

What are the new responsibilities of the clinician who must continue to remain focused on the needs and demands of an individual patient but must also take account of patients not yet in contact with the service?

How do these new responsibilities relate to the traditional responsibility of doctors?

■ The changing contractual position of doctors

In the 20th century, it was argued that the doctor's responsibilities were to the individual patient in a consultation and to that patient alone. Until 1948, doctors in the United Kingdom received their income directly from the patient sitting in front of them. This simple contractual arrangement is shown in Figure 1.1. For doctors in some other countries, this is still the contractual position today.

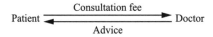

Figure 1.1 The 'direct' contractual arrangement between doctor and patient

However, with the founding of the National Health Service (NHS), the contractual relationship between doctors and patients changed (see Figure 1.2). People were no longer prevented from accessing care by its cost because the resources for care were provided by the whole population. Within the population providing

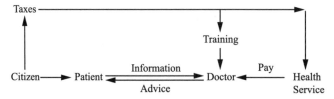

Figure 1.2 The new contractual relationship between doctors and patients

■ 从资源中获取更多价值

虽然医生的时间有限，但是可以通过诸如拓展在线咨询等形式来增加面对面沟通的时间，从而带来获益。金钱也是有限的，但与时间不同，不能通过其他方式进行扩展和增加。金钱同样缺乏灵活性：为一名患者所花的费用不能再转移到另一名患者身上。因此，如果要使已经满负荷运转的医疗系统服务更多的人群，就需要从现有资源中获取更多价值。这是新挑战，也势必成为临床医生的新职责。

临床医生必须继续关注个体患者的需要和需求，但也必须同时关注那些还没有享受卫生服务的患者。在这种情况下，临床医生新的职责是什么？

这些新职责与医生的传统职责有什么关系？

■ 医患合同关系的不断变化

在20世纪，医生的职责只针对个体患者，而且只需要对诊治的患者负责即可。1948年以前，英国医生直接向诊治的患者收费。图1.1展示了这种简单的合同关系。某些国家仍在沿用这种医患合同关系。

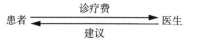

图1.1　医生和患者之间的"直接"合同关系

然而，随着英国国家卫生服务体系（National Health Service，NHS）的建立，医患之间的合同关系已经发生了变化（图1.2）。患者不再因无法承担医疗费用而无法获得医治，因为卫生服务是由全民买单。为这些医疗资源买

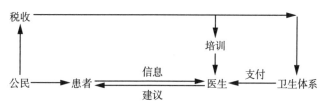

图1.2　医生和患者之间的新型合同关系

the resources for care, some people：

- *are patients already in contact with the service*;
- *have the condition (i.e. are in need) but have not yet made contact with the service*;
- *are healthy and will never develop the condition (i.e. not in need)*.

With the exception of the United States of America, this contractual arrangement exists in every developed country, although it is possible that the USA is now on the way to complete coverage of its population.

However, in the NHS, this change in contractual arrangement had disadvantages. Some doctors no longer acted as if the 'customer was king' and treated patients with less respect.

Few doctors regarded themselves as the stewards of NHS resources and acted merely as the dispensers of resources. One medical manager remarked：'it is as if doctors were writing a cheque in the supermarket but thought that their bank was going to pay, not their own account. '

■ Medical management-responsibility and accountability for a service

In the last decade of the 20th century, new responsibilities for doctors were articulated-responsibilities for patient safety, quality of care, and resource management. However, many clinicians were unwilling to accept the responsibility for managing resources, leaving only a small proportion of clinicians to become medical managers. Of those clinicians who accepted the role, most were part-time; however, some became full-time medical directors or chief executives of a hospital (see Figure 1.3).

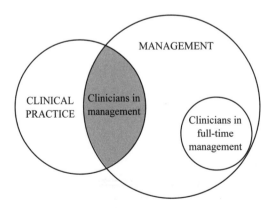

Figure 1.3 The relationship of clinicians to resource management

单的人群包括：

- 已经使用医疗卫生保健的患者；

- 有需要但尚未使用卫生服务资源的人；

- 现在健康，且永远不会患这种病的人（即，无需求者）。

除美国外，所有发达国家都存在这种合同契约，但是美国现在也在尝试改革，让这种合同契约逐步覆盖全部人口。

然而在NHS中，合同契约的改变引起很多问题。一些医生不再遵循"顾客是上帝"的原则，对患者变得不够尊重。

很少有医生自视其为公共资源的管理者，而仅承担着医疗资源提供者的角色。一位医疗管理者描述，"这就好比医生在超市里开支票，他们认为这钱是由银行来支付而不是花自己账户上的钱"。

■ 医疗管理——服务的职责与义务

在20世纪最后10年里，患者安全、医疗质量和资源管理被明确纳入临床医生的职责范畴。然而，只有一小部分临床医生成为医疗管理者，大多数临床医生不愿承担资源管理的责任。在接受了管理者角色的临床医生中，大多数人以兼职身份同时开展临床实践与资源管理，但是也有一部分临床医生成为专职医疗主管或医院的首席执行官（图1.3）。

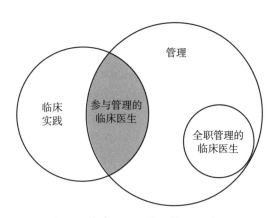

图1.3　临床医生和资源管理的关系

■ Population medicine-accountability to and for a population

In the 21st century, the responsibilities of a doctor continue to include loyalty and commitment to the well-being of an individual patient and to the quality and safety of the care they provide. However, these responsibilities are now complemented and supplemented by a new responsibility, a responsibility to the population that provides the resources for care.

The population providing the resources for care contains the patients who are already being treated, but for every long-term condition it also includes other people with the condition who have not yet been referred. Furthermore, the population which made the decision to allocate the resources for healthcare has done so having decided that those resources will produce more value from healthcare than if they were invested in education, state pensions, defence, or any other public service.

With resources always being limited, by choosing to implement one option, there is a benefit forgone as resources are then not available for other options. The lost benefit from the next best use of the resources is the opportunity cost. (1)

The good management of resources by a medical manager is of obvious benefit to the population but population medicine entails more than resource management. Clinicians in the 21st century are expected to act as the stewards of the allocated resources, and to become conscious not only of the people who could benefit from healthcare or who are already in receipt of this benefit, but also of the 'benefit foregone' by the whole population such as the education of children or the amelioration of poverty.

The concept of stewardship has a long history: originally it concerned the administration of an estate on behalf of the lord of the manor. More recently, the concept carries connotations of a deeper responsibility that has arisen from its use in the context of environmental sustainability, for example:

Stewardship is to hold something in trust for another. (2)
The stewardship concept demands that we constantly ask the question: will the resource be in better shape after my stewardship? (3)

■ 群医学——为人群健康承担责任

在21世纪，临床医生的职责仍然包括全心全意治疗每个患者、以患者福祉为己任，为他们提供安全合格的卫生保健服务。但是现在这些已经被新职责所补充完善，即需要对全人群提供医疗卫生保健资源。

临床医生既需要为已在接受治疗和长期有卫生服务需求的患者提供资源，也需要为没有转诊到卫生服务体系接受服务的患者提供资源。此外，那些决定将资源分配给医疗卫生保健的民众认为，与投资教育、养老、国防或者任何其他公共服务相比，将这些资源投入医疗卫生保健服务会获取更大的价值。

资源总是有限的，选择将资源投入一个领域，其他领域就无法利用这笔资源了，这样就会造成收益损失。在投资决策中，放弃次优方案而损失的潜在利益，就是选取最优方案的机会成本。[1]

医疗管理者如果能够很好地管理资源，会明显改善人群健康的效益；但是，群医学对资源管理者的要求却并非止步于此。21世纪的临床医生应该成为真正意义的资源管理者——"资源管家"（stewards）——他们不仅要了解谁将会从卫生保健中获益，谁已经获益；还需要认识到将资源分配给医疗卫生领域的机会成本，如未投资儿童教育、消除贫困等方面损失的潜在利益（benefit foregone）。

"管家职权"（stewardship）的概念有悠久的历史：起初这个词主要表示代表庄园主管理庄园的工作。现在，这个概念在可持续发展背景下，衍生出更深层次的责任：

"管家职权"就是受他人委托掌管某物。[2]

"管家职权"的理念要求我们不断地问这样一个问题：我的"管家职权"是否优化了资源分配？[3]

In parallel with calls for a broader perspective to be taken in clinical practice, one that takes into account not only the patient's clinical condition-personalisation — but also the patient's values and the environment in which they live-contextualisation — a broader perspective is required when considering a health service with responsibility for and accountability to not only the patients in contact with the service-the traditional role of the clinician as medical manager-but also the whole population of people in need, as well as an accountability to the population that has provided the resources for care (Figure 1.4).

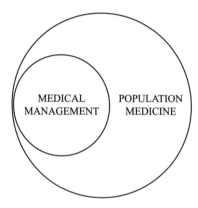

Figure 1.4 Population medicine embraces medical management

■ Seven actions to improve the health of populations

In the first decade of the 21st century, the focus of management and leadership development has been on managing an institution, either a health centre or a hospital. The emphasis on quality improvement, on making care more effective, and on safety (see Box 1.1), also focused around institutions, has been essential, but it is not sufficient to meet the challenges of the 21st century.

Clinicians of the 21st century have a responsibility not just to the patients who happen to have made contact with their service but also for all the people whose needs could be met, directly or indirectly, by their service. In addition to achieving high levels of quality and safety, there are seven actions that need to be taken to discharge this new set of responsibilities and improve the health of populations (see Table 1.1).

现在都在呼吁从更广阔的视角审视临床实践，这不仅要考虑患者个体的临床状态（个性化），也要考虑患者的价值观和他们的生活背景（情景化）。同时，采用更广阔的视角考虑医疗卫生保健时，需要临床医生承担作为医疗管理者的传统责任，为已进入卫生系统内的个体患者提供良好的医疗照护，还应当让所有有医疗需求的人能够利用好卫生资源（图1.4）。况且，医疗资源本由全人群提供，也必须为全人群尽责。

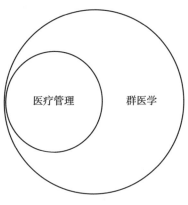

图1.4　群医学包括医疗管理

■ 提升人群健康水平的七大行动

在21世纪的前10年，关于管理和领导力开发的研究多聚焦于如何管理一家机构，例如一家健康照护中心或者医院。以这些机构为中心，着重关注如何持续改进医疗质量，确保医疗安全且更加高效，这些依然是不可或缺的（专栏1.1），却已不足以应对21世纪的诸多挑战。

21世纪临床医生的职责不仅是为那些主动寻求医疗照护的患者人群提供帮助，而且还应尽其所能满足所有人群直接或间接的健康服务医疗需求。除了不懈追求优质安全的医疗照护外，还需要采取七大行动来履行一系列的新职责，寻求改善人群的整体健康水平（表1.1）。

Box 1.1 The Better Value Healthcare Bookshop

In the Better Value Healthcare Bookshop[1], there are more than 30 books on safety and about 100 books on quality improvement. For medical management, these books are essential; for population medicine, they are necessary but not sufficient because this approach necessitates many actions other than those relating to the delivery of services to higher standards of quality and safety. Key texts for each topic are listed below.

Books on safety
Patient Safety by Charles Vincent
Understanding Patient Safety by Robert Wachter

Books on the theory of medical errors and accidents
The Human Contribution by James Reason
Complications by Atul Gawande
Safety and Ethics in Healthcare by Bill Runciman

Books on quality improvement
The classic remains *An Introduction to Quality Assurance in Health Care* by Avedis Donabedian. Some books focus solely on healthcare, such as *Quality by Design: A Clinical Microsystem Approach* by Eugene Nelson, Paul Batalden and Marjorie Godfrey.

The majority describe quality improvement and quality assurance in industry, particularly in Japanese industry and, within that, at Toyota.

Table 1.1 Discharging new responsibilities for improving population health in the 21st century

New responsibility	Action
Value	Getting the right patients to the right resources
Outcomes	Getting the right outcomes for the right patients
Waste	Getting the right outcomes with the least waste
Sustainability	Doing the right things to protect resources for future generations
Equity	Ensuring fairness and justice
Supporting all patients, not just those referred	Creating populationg-based, integrated systems
Health promotion	Preventing disease and promoting health and well-being

---

[1] http://astore.amazon.co.uk/betterv-21

专栏 1.1 卫生保健价值优选书目（附网址[1]）

在这个主题书店里，有超过30本介绍医疗安全的著作和大约100本阐述质量改进的著作。对于医疗管理实践，这些书籍是必备的；而就群医学实践而言，这些书籍同样必要但并不够。因为要做好群医学实践，除了完成那些以更高的质量和安全标准提供的医疗服务外，还需要采取许多其他的行动。以下所列就是关于上述主题的一些重要原著。

1. 有关安全性的著作
《患者安全》 查尔斯·文森特著
《领悟患者安全》 罗伯特·沃克特著

2. 关于医疗差错和医疗事故的理论著作
《人类的贡献》 詹姆斯·里曾著
《并发症》 阿图尔·加万德著
《卫生保健的安全与伦理》 比尔·朗西曼著

3. 关于质量改进的著作
堪称经典的《质量保证概述》 阿维迪斯·多纳贝迪安著
有些著作仅重点关注卫生保健，例如《设计质量：一种临床微系统路径》 尤金·纳尔逊、保罗·巴塔登和马乔里·戈弗雷著

大多数著作描述工业领域中的质量改进和质量保证，尤其关于日本工业界，其中包括丰田公司。

表 1.1 21世纪为促进人群健康水平所应履行的新职责

新职责	行动目标
价值	让合适的患者都能获得合适的资源
结局	让合适的患者都能得到合适的结局
避免浪费	以最少的浪费追求合适的结果
可持续	做正确的事，保护资源，以利后人
公平	确保公平与公正
为所有患者提供支持，而不仅是就医者	构建基于人群的整合型体系
健康促进	预防疾病，促进健康与福祉

[1] http://astore.amazon.co.uk/betterv-21

The first three of these responsibilities could be seen as an extension of the clinician's responsibility to the organisation that employs them, but the latter four, which are inter-related, are completely new. Of these new responsibilities, perhaps the most challenging is the commitment to all people in need, and not just to those people who have been referred.

From one perspective, broken legs do not pose a problem for health services. All the people with broken legs reach the right service, irrespective of the assertiveness of the patient, the patient's social status or the competence and beliefs of a general practitioner. People with cancer also tend to reach the right service, although there may be delays in the time taken to reach the service due to factors relating to the beliefs and behaviours of both patients and clinicians. For people who have one or more long-term conditions, however, many of them who could benefit from the knowledge and skills of specialist services do not because they are not referred (see Figure 1.5). This problem is common for this group of patients.

There are three possible solutions to this problem.

1. Expand the specialist service, but this is rarely possible in an era of constraint.

2. Clarify and implement referral criteria to reduce the size of the problem as depicted in Figure 1.5.

3. Change the way of working in the specialist service such that the knowl-

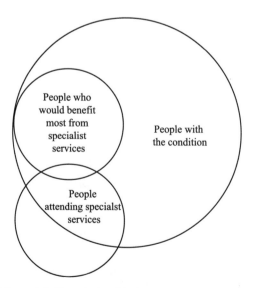

People who would benefit most from specialist services

People with the condition

People attending specialst services

Figure 1.5 The relationship between need and supply

这7大职责中的前3项职责，可看做是医生对其岗位职责的延伸，但是后四项是内在相互关联而且是全新的职责。对于这些全新的职责，也许最大的挑战是对"所有有需求的群体"而不仅是对那些"前来求医者"负责。

从某种意义上，腿部骨折不会对医疗卫生保健系统造成麻烦。因为所有腿部骨折患者都能得到妥善救治，而这与患者的个人决断能力、社会地位或者全科医生自己的能力和信仰等关系不大。癌症患者也在一定程度上能得到妥善救治，但受到患者本人和救治医生的信仰及行为等相关因素的影响，患者有可能并没有得到及时救治。然而，对于长期患有一种或多种疾病的人来说，他们中有很多人本来有可能从专科医生的知识和技能照护中受益，但由于他们没能被及时转诊，而最终没有获益（图1.5），此类问题在长期患病者群中很常见。

此类问题有3种可能的解决方案：

1. 扩大专科诊疗范围，但是在一个资源稀缺的时代，这种可能性很小。

2. 明确并实施精准的转诊标准，以减少图1.5所描述问题的规模。

3. 改变专科医生的工作方式，以便专科知识和技能可以直接或间接地

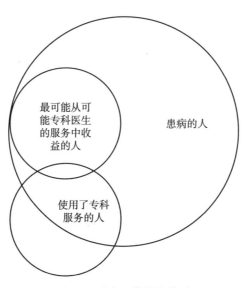

图1.5　需求和供给的关系

edge and skills of the specialists can be made available, either directly or indirectly, to all the patients who could benefit (i.e. all those in need), which is likely to be a much larger number than those currently being seen by the specialist service; at present, specialist service resources at present can be accessed only by a patient visiting healthcare real estate.

The changes outlined in point 3 above need to be delivered by clinicians working according to the new paradigm, known as 'population medicine'.

■ What is different about population medicine?

Population medicine is a style of clinical practice or a way of working. It does not replace other paradigms, such as evidence-based medicine or patient-centered care, but instead it complements and supplements them. When clinicians practising population medicine see individual patients, they continue to use best current evidence and be patient-centred, but they also need to address the root causes of failures in the quality of care. This is best demonstrated by considering the questions clinicians might ask themselves while reflecting on the day's clinic (see Display 1.1).

Display 1.1 A traditional and a population approach to resolving the problems posed by the presentation of a child with asthma

Scenario: A child with asthma whose problems shoud have been able to be managed by the child, and the child's family and general practitioner	
Clinician restricted to the traditional responsibilities in healthcare	*Clinician fulfilling the responsibilities of population medicine*
● Why did the child not know how to use her spacer? ● Why did the general practitioner refer the child when it would have been possible to resolve the problem using the local clinical guidelines?	● Why was the general practitioner (GP) not able to manage the child without referral? *Because the GP did not follow the guidelines.* ● Why did the GP not follow the guidelines? *Because the GP did not know of their existence.* ● Why did the GP not know of the existence of the guidelines? *Because the GP was new to the area.* ● Why are new GPs not informed about the existence of guidelines? *Because we have no system for identifying and informing new GPs.* ● Why do we not set up a process to identify new GPs and pharmacists to ensure they know about local guidelines, resources and referral protocols?

使所有患者（当需要时）受益；如是，其数量可能远大于目前专科医生所能照护的人数。目前，患者只有前往医疗机构就诊才能接触到各种专科医疗照护资源。

要想做到第3点，临床医生就要考虑根据群医学实施新的范式。

■ 群医学有何不同？

群医学是一种临床实践形式或一种工作方式。群医学并非要取代其他工作范式，如基于循证医学的实践或以患者为中心的医疗照护，而是对这些工作范式进行补充与完善。当医生以群医学视角去面对个体患者时，他们依旧要应用当前最佳的证据，以患者为中心开展诊疗活动，但是他们也需要透过对个体患者的照护，找出医疗质量没有得到保证的根本原因，最好的实践方法就是临床医生每天回顾和反思自己日常临床工作中遇到的问题，见场景1.1。

场景1.1　在解决儿童哮喘问题时，传统的医学
和群医学的差异

情况：一个哮喘患儿，他的症状本应由该儿童、儿童的家庭和全科医生共同解决	
在医疗中坚守传统的医学职责的医生	履行群医学职责的医生
● 为什么这个儿童不知道如何使用储雾罐？ ● 一个使用本地临床指南就可以解决的问题，为什么全科医生要把这个孩子转诊？	● 为什么全科医生在不转诊的情况下，不能对该儿童哮喘实施有效的管理？因为该全科医生没有遵循相关指南 ● 为什么该全科医生没有遵循指南？因为全科医生不知道该指南的存在 ● 为什么该全科医生不知道指南的存在？因为该全科医生是这个地区的新从业者 ● 为什么没有人告知该全科医生指南的存在？因为我们没有识别新入职全科医生并告知其相关信息的系统 ● 为什么我们不建立一个可以识别新入职的全科医生及药剂师的系统，以确保他们能够了解当地指南、资源和转诊的程序？

The clinician with a traditional approach asks a different set of questions from that posed by the clinician with a population medicine perspective, which is based on the 'Five Whys' approach developed by the Toyota Motor Corporation.

The population medicine approach answers Question 5 by putting in place the necessary systems to prevent a recurrence of the problem. Another approach using the Five Whys as a foundation would be to ask a different set of questions than the simple rhetorical question, 'Why did the child not know how to use her spacer?' (see Display 1.2). Here are eight questions that a clinician practising population medicine could ask.

Display 1.2 A populaion approach to the root causes of why children with asthma do not have the knowledge for good self-management

Scenario: A child with asthma who does not know how to use their spacer
1. How many children are there with asthma in the local population?
2. What poportion of children is referred to the specialist service?
3. How many are referred to could be managed by generalists, such as GPs and pharmacists?
4. How many children to should be referred are not?
5. Are we clear about our objectives, guidelines and referral criteria?
6. Are all the generalists working with the local population including those most newly appointed aware of our guidelines and referral criteria?
7. Are all the people with asthma and their carers fully informed about how they can best manage their condition?
8. How good is the service for the local population when compared with services for similar populations in other localities?

From a bureaucratic perspective, the components of a typical health service could be represented as a set of interconnected but separate boxes(see Figure 1.6).

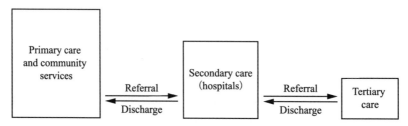

Figure 1.6 The traditional model of institutionalised care

以群医学为视角的临床医生可以基于丰田汽车公司开发的"五个为什么"工具提出一系列问题。这些问题与采用传统模式的临床医生提出问题有所不同。

群医学通过建立必要的体系，解决第五个问题，防止类似情形再次发生。再举一个使用"五个为什么"方法的例子。可提出一组不同的问题，而不仅是用一个简单的设问句，例如：为什么儿童不知道如何使用储雾罐？（场景1.2）下面列举了一个临床医生从群医学的视角可能问到的8个问题。

场景1.2 以群医学视角探索哮喘患儿及其家庭缺乏足够
自我管理知识的根本原因

情景：哮喘患儿及其家庭不知道如何使用储雾罐
● 当地人口中有多少儿童患有哮喘？
● 有多大比例的儿童被转诊到专科进行治疗？
● 被转诊的儿童有多少可以由通科医生，如全科医生、药剂师进行有效管理？
● 有多少儿童应当被转诊而实际并没有转诊？
● 我们是否清楚治疗目标、指南和转诊标准？
● 是不是所有的全科医生（包括新入职的）都清楚指南和转诊标准？
● 是否所有的哮喘患者及其照料者都被告知应当如何管理他们的病情？
● 与其他地区的相似群体相比，本地区医疗服务质量如何？

从行政程序角度看，典型的医疗服务组成部分可由一组相互关联但又相互独立的单元表示（图1.6）。

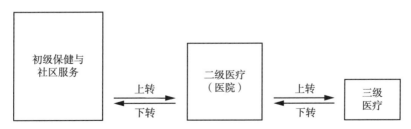

图1.6 医疗机构患者管理的传统模式

However, there are several mis-representations regarding the depiction of reality in this figure; in reality:

- *there are large overlaps between primary and secondary care services, and between secondary and tertiary care services;*
- *a hospital is portrayed as being different and distinct from 'community' services, but this perpetuates the myth that a hospital is not a community service (1).*

Another way to depict the relationship of the different types of care is as a Venn diagram (Figure 1.3), in which the different types of care are shown as a set of nested boxes, referred to as 'four-box' healthcare.

An individual may make use of all four types of care during the course of a year, or even a day; as can be seen from Figure 1.7, there are 'passages' from one type of care to another. 'Five-box' healthcare is shown in Figure 1.8, revealing the relationship when super-specialist care (e.g. a paediatric neurology service) is included. The passage from generalist care to specialist care has a filter, as does the passage from specialist care to super-specialist care.

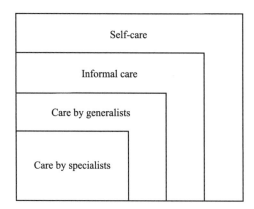

Figure 1.7　'Four-box' healthcare

The concept of filters was developed in one of the first books on healthcare systems — *Mental Illness in the Community: Pathways to Psychiatric Care* (4). In this book, several levels of service provision in mental health services were identified together with a filter between each level, as shown Box 1.2. The match between need and resources in mental health services was clearly described and found to be far from perfect.

然而，这幅示意图不是对现实情况的准确描述。现实的情况是：

- 在初级和二级、二级和三级医疗服务之间，都存在着大量重叠。
- 人们一般都认为，医院与"社区"提供的医疗服务是有区别的，这使得"医院不属于社区医疗服务"这一观念根深蒂固[1]。

一种描述不同类型医疗卫生保健之间关系的方法是用维恩图（图1.7），图中不同类型的医疗卫生保健用一组嵌套的盒子表示，被称为"四层式"医疗卫生保健。

一个人可以在一年甚至一天内使用4种类型的医疗卫生保健服务，如图1.7所示，而且不同类型的医疗卫生保健之间都有联结通道。图1.8展示了"五层式"医疗保健，揭示了包含亚专科医生提供的健康保健医疗照护（如小儿神经科服务）在内的关系。从全科照护到专科照护的转化是经过筛选的，同样从专科照护到亚专科照护也是如此。

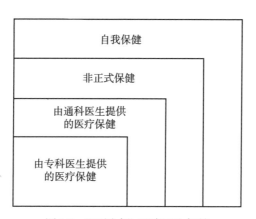

图1.7　"四层式"医疗卫生保健

筛选路径的概念是在第一批关于卫生系统书籍之一——《社区中的精神疾病：精神疾病保健路径》中提出的[4]。该书确定了提供精神卫生服务提供的层级，并在每个层级之间进行了筛选，如专栏1.2所示。专栏清楚阐述了心理健康服务的需求和资源之间的匹配，但匹配程度远不完善。

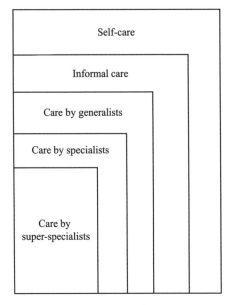

Figure 1.8 'Five-box' healthcare

Box 1.2 Levels of service provision and filters in mental health services (4)

Psychiatrically ill during the year.

FILTER 1: the person's belief about the nature of their problem-e.g. is it normal grief or clinical depression.

Consult their doctor during the year.

FILTER 2: their relationship with their general practitioner and the ease of access.

Recognised as psychiatrically ill by their doctor.

FILTER 3: the generalist's skills.

Referred to a specialist service.

FILTER 4: the generalist's knowledge and beliefs, and the ease of access to the specialist service.

Admitted to a specialist service.

■ Generalist and specialist partnerships

There is an increasing recognition both implicitly and explicitly that clinicians have responsibilities to the whole population as well as to the individual patient. Although general practitioners have practiced population medicine since 1948, when each was allocated a defined population for which they were responsible, and hospital specialists have had some population responsibilities to which they have responded to varying degrees, some recent trends in healthcare management in the NHS, such as the development of Foundation Trusts, have mitigated against the exercise of responsibility for populations.

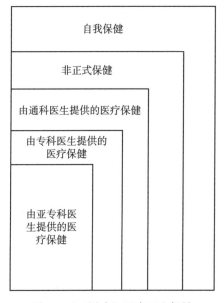

图1.8 "五层式"医疗卫生保健

专栏1.2 精神卫生服务的层级和筛选路径[4]

这一年精神疾病的患病情况

筛选路径1：本人对问题本质的认知，例如是正常状态的悲伤情绪还是临床上的抑郁表现。

在年内咨询其医生

筛选路径2：他们与全科医生的关系及其可及性。

被医生诊断为患有精神疾病

筛选路径3：全科医生的各项技能。

转诊到专科医生

筛选路径4：全科医生的知识与信念，以及转诊到专科医生的可及性。

进入专科服务

■ 全科医生与专科医生的伙伴关系

人们越来越清楚地认识到，临床医生对整个人群和患者个人都负有责任。虽然自1948年全科医生开始从事群医学，当时每名全科医生都需要负责特定人群，在医院工作的专科医生也承担特定人群的医疗照护，并且对人群的不同状态进行分级，然而，近年来NHS医疗管理的一些趋势，比如信托基金的发展，弱化了医生对人群健康的责任。

The relationship between generalists and specialists is often unnecessarily fraught for two reasons.

1. Many members of both types of practitioner fail to understand the difference between the sensitivity of a symptom, sign or test result and its positive predictive value. In general practice, where the incidence and prevalence of disease is lower, the implications of the presence of a symptom, sign or positive test result is of much less concern than in specialist practice where the incidence and prevalence of the disease is much higher, principally because the generalists only refer those patients who obviously have the disease or who have a high probability of having the disease. This leads specialists to criticise generalists for missing 'easy' diagnoses and generalists to criticise specialists for over-investigation.

2. There is an important difference between complex and complicated medical problems. A complex problem is epitomised by an 80-year-old woman with four diagnoses and seven prescriptions, looked after by her 50-year-old daughter who has an alcoholic husband and an unemployed son. This type of situation is standard in general practice. However, when one of the diagnosed diseases becomes complicated, such as heart failure developing in the Parkinson's disease, the generalist seeks specialist help.

To maximise value for the population, it is important:

- *To help generalists and specialists work together*;
- *To recognise the need to use the knowledge and skills of specialists to serve the patients in the population who have not been referred in addition to the patients who have been referred to them*;
- *To encourage and fund specialists to apply their knowledge and skills to the care of the population in need*.

Ways in which value for the population in need can be maximised by hospital specialists working in partnership with generalists are shown in Display 1.3. It is important to emphasise that the specialist or consultant with responsibility for a population does not become responsible for every patient.

全科医生与专科医生的关系经常引起无端的困扰，其原因有以下两点：

1. 很多全科医生和专科医生都未能理解症状、体征或检测结果的灵敏度与其阳性预测值之间的区别。在全科诊疗中，就诊人员的发病率和患病率较低。其症状、体征或阳性检测结果的影响要比在专科诊疗中小得多；全科医生通常将那些明显患病或患病概率更高的人转诊给专科医生。因此，专科就诊人员的发病率和患病率更高。所以，全科医生对症状、体征或检测结果的关注度远低于专科医生。这种情况导致专科医生经常批评全科医生漏诊那些"显而易见"的诊断，而全科医生则抱怨专科医生对患者过度检查。

2. 医疗问题的复合性（complex）和复杂性（complicated）是两个不同的概念。这里举例说明医疗问题的复合性：一位80岁的老太太，患有4种疾病且需要接受7种处方的治疗，由自己50岁的女儿照料；而她50岁的女儿又有一个酗酒的丈夫和一个无职业的儿子。这种情况在全科医生工作中很常见。然而，当某种已被确诊的疾病恶化时，就出现了问题的复杂性，如一个帕金森患者出现了心力衰竭，此时全科医生就需要寻求专科医生的帮助。

为了实现医疗卫生保健对人群价值的最大化，重要的是：

● 帮助促进全科医生和专科医生通力合作；

● 认识到专科医生的知识和技能不仅要用于被转诊来的患者，也要用于没有被转诊来的患者；

● 鼓励并资助专科医生运用自己的知识和技能服务于有需求的人群。

场景1.3展示了全科医生和专科医生合作以最大限度地满足人群需求的方法。需要强调的是，对人群负责的专科医生或顾问并不意味着需要对每一个患者负责。

Display 1.3 Specialists and generalists working in partnership to take a population approach to COPD

Scenario: A specialist service for COPD at which 800 patients a year are seen by the consultant in respiratory medicine
• Specialist service to estimate the number of patients with COPD in the population covered by the clinical networks in which the consultant works, based on published epidemiological studies and prescribing data (~2000)
• Conduct an audit across the clinical networks to identify people who have not been referred but who would benefit from referral (~200)
• Hold a joint discussion about how to increase productivity: whether the specialist service should see 1000 extra patients a year using the same level of resources or whether general practitioners manage 200 of the 800 people referred if GPs are given more support by the specialist service
• Specialist service to identify, through an analysis of prescribing and referral patterns, the scope for the specialist service to give greater support to certain general practitioners
• Specialist service to ensure that important new evidence reaches all those healthcare professionals who need to be aware of it
• Specialist service to ensure that all people with COPD receive unbiased information
• Specialist service to accept responsibility for the local variant of the Map of Medicine®
• Specialist service to take responsibility for the professional development of all general practitioners, physiotherapists and pharmacists who are seeing patients with COPD in the population covered by the network
• Specialist service to coordinate and lead the network of all relevant professionals and patient organisations
• Specialist service to produce an annual report

The generalist (family doctor, primary care physician or general practitioner) retains responsibility for the patients who are registered with them. Nor does the specialist become responsible for the clinical care of all the individuals in a population. However, they do become responsible for the health of all the people who have the condition about which they have specialist knowledge, and all the people who might develop it (i.e. those who are or could be in need). Thus, they are also responsible not just for the quality and value of care delivered for people with the relevant condition, but also for the prevention of that condition and for helping people with that condition lead a full and healthy life.

To enable clinicians to fulfil all the responsibilities of population medicine:

- *these responsibilities need to be recognised in clinicians' job descriptions*;
- *time should be allocated to enable clinicians to carry out these responsibilities, perhaps one day a week.*

场景 1.3　全科医生和专科医生合作，以群医学的工作方式
应对慢性阻塞性肺疾病

> 情景：每年由呼吸科专家为800名慢性阻塞性肺疾病患者提供专科医疗照顾
>
> - 专科医生基于已发表的流行病学研究和处方数据，估算临床工作网络中的慢性阻塞性肺疾病的患者数量（约2000名）
> - 在临床网络上审核那些应该转诊但没有转诊的患者（约200名）
> - 全科医生与专科医生一同讨论如何提高体系效率：在使用同样卫生资源的情况下，专科医生在一年内是否有能力多服务1000名患者，或全科医生在专科医生更多的帮助下，是否能仅转诊800名患者中的200名
> - 通过对处方和转诊模式展开分析，确定专科医生可以在多大程度上给予某些全科医生更大的支持
> - 专科医生需确保那些有必要知晓最新循证信息的医疗卫生保健专业人员能够获得这些信息
> - 专科医生需要确保所有慢性阻塞性肺疾病患者获得准确无误的信息
> - 当医疗片区的划分有变动时，专科医生承担相应的职责
> - 专科医生应该帮助全科医生、物理治疗师和药剂师提高专业素质，以服务那些工作网络覆盖人群中的慢性阻塞性肺疾病患者
> - 专科医生需要协调和领导工作网络内所有的专业人员和患者团体
> - 此项专科服务每年生成一份年度报告

通科医生（又称家庭医生、初级卫生保健医生或全科医生）仍需要对在他们名下登记在册的患者负责，而专科医生不需要对人群中每个个体的临床照护负责。然而，由于专科医生掌握了某种疾病的专业知识，他们也的确需要对所有患有这种疾病的人以及将来可能患这种疾病的人（即那些需要或可能需要帮助的人）的健康负责。因此，他们不仅要为相关疾病患者提供质量合格的医疗卫生保健服务，还要负责预防此类疾病发生，并帮助患者安享充实健康的生活。

为了让临床医生能够履行群医学的全部职责：

- 需要把上述职责纳入到临床医生的岗位职责描述中；
- 需要给临床医生一定的时间以履行这些职责，比如一周一天。

However, the lead consultant may also require support for the coordination of the network, with help from a clinical scientist or administrator. A job description with key responsibilities for the clinician who takes the leading role for population medicine is set out in Display 1.4, although it is not envisaged that many clinicians will be full-time in population medicine.

Display 1.4 Job description for a lead clinician with responsibility for population medicine, taking neurological disease as an example

Aim	● To improve the health of all the people with neurological disease in the local population served
Key result areas	● To promote the prevention of neurological disease ● To develop and maintain estimates of the total numbers of people with common neurological disease and problems ● For each common neurological disease, to ensure that there is a system of care with appropriate criteria and standards with each system expressed as a care pathway ● To build and sustain a clinical network ● To work with patients and their representatives to help people with neurological disease to participate as partners in their care and to live a full life and have a good death ● To promote research ● To produce an annual report for the population served
Resources	The post-holder will have one day a week reserved for this work. They will be supported by an information scientist with knowledge management skills working two days a week and have a small budget to facilitate their work
Key relationships	● Local branches of relevant patient groups ● Local branches of relevant professional associations ● Public health professionals serving the population ● Relevant managers and policy-makers

■ The ethical issues of population medicine

When the topic of population medicine is first raised, some clinicians will be concerned about the potential ethical conflict, as they perceive it, between their total commitment to the individual patient and an explicit responsibility to the population. However, clinicians have always had to manage that most precious of resources, their time, not only by considering what the patient in front of them wants but also the needs of other patients. Although many patients would like more of the clinician's time, all clinicians have to consider how best to use this finite resource.

然而，主管的专科医生可能仍需行政人员和临床科研人员协助开展工作网络。场景1.4 列举了主管群医学工作的临床医生的岗位描述和主要职责，但这并不意味着很多临床医生将全职从事群医学工作。

场景1.4 主管群医学的临床医生岗位职责描述
——以神经医学为例

目的	● 提高服务地区人群神经系统疾病患者的健康水平
达成的关键结果	● 促进神经系统疾病的预防 ● 动态监测该地区常见神经系统疾病的患者以及有相关困扰者的人数 ● 对每一种常见的神经系统疾病，建立包括适宜的标准和规范在内的系统管理，每一体系都以工作路径展现 ● 建立并维持临床工作网络 ● 与患者及其代理人合作，帮助神经系统疾病患者参与自身护理，过上充实生活、安详离世 ● 推动相关研究 ● 为服务人群提供一份年度报告
资源	● 负责该岗位的医生每周预留一天时间从事本项（群医学）工作。那些具有知识管理技能的信息学专家则每周用两天时间为其提供帮助，也需要一点资金以支持他们更好地开展工作
核心关系	● 相关患者组织在当地的分支机构 ● 相关专业协会在地方的分支机构 ● 为人群服务的公共卫生专业人员 ● 相关管理人员和政策制定者

■ 群医学的伦理问题

群医学首次被提出时，一些临床医生担心：在他们对个体患者的承诺和对人群的明确责任之间存在潜在的伦理冲突。实际上，临床医生总是不得不管理他们最宝贵的资源——时间，他们不仅要考虑他们面前的患者需要什么，还要考虑其他患者的需求。虽然许多患者都希望临床医生在提供医疗照护时能够付出更多的时间，但是所有临床医生都必须考虑如何最好地使用这种有限的时间资源。

However, in a situation where clinicians have to make judgements about whether to allocate additional financial resources to the patient in front of them, this does present an ethical problem. The problem can be prevented by ensuring that decisions on the allocation of resources are not made by the individual clinician during a consultation, but through a process that is open and accountable. Daniels and Sabin have expounded the type of accountability necessary for such decision-making.

Accountability for reasonableness is the idea that the reasons or rationales for important limit-setting decisions should be publicly available. In addition, these reasons must be ones that 'fair-minded' people can agree are relevant to pursuing appropriate patient care under necessary resource constraints. This is our central thesis, and it needs some explanation.

By 'fair-minded', we do not simply mean our friends or people who just happen to agree with us. We mean people who in principle seek to cooperate with others on terms they can justify to each other. Indeed, fair-minded people accept rules of the game — or sometimes seek rule changes — that promote the game's essential skills and the excitement their use produces. (5)

At the beginning of the 21st century, an increasing number of people would agree that it is now unethical not to consider the whole population as well as the individual patient. The principal argument in the debate is about environmental change and resource use, as opposed to lower-value healthcare. These environmental issues, however, are highly relevant and relate to the phenomenon known as 'the tragedy of the commons' in which environmental degradation occurs whenever many individuals use a scarce resource in common (see Display 1.5). Reuben argues that this is the situation in healthcare (6). If every clinician and every patient uses more and more of the finite healthcare resources, there will come a point when the health service breaks down and everyone suffers.

Display 1.5 The tragedy of the commons

Scenario: Imagine you are a farmer grazing your sheep on common land
Custom and tradition mean that you are allowed to have 20 sheep on the common land, but you introduce one more and no-one seems to notice or mind. So the next year you introduce another sheep, and the following year another, and so on. Unfortunately, all the other commoners have adopted the same policy such that a point is reached when the whole ecosystem collapses, the grass does not grow and all the sheep die. This is the tragedy of the commons.

然而，在临床医生必须判断是否应该为面前患者分配额外的财政资源时，确实面临伦理问题。要想避免这一问题，就需要确保资源配置决策过程是公开和可信的，而不是由某个临床医生在提供就诊咨询服务期间擅自决定。丹尼尔斯（Daniels）和萨宾（Sabin）阐述了此类决策所需的责任类型。

合理性问责是指应该公开重要的资源限制决策的理由或依据。此外，这些理由必须是那些"公正的"人们能够认同的，与在必要的资源限制下寻求适当的患者照护有关。这是我们的中心论题而且需要加以解释。

我们所说的"公正的"人并不是简单指我们的朋友或恰好与我们意见一致的人，而是那些原则上寻求与他人合作的人，他们可以向对方证明自己的理由。事实上，有公平意识的人接受行业规则——或者有时寻求规则改变——以提升行业所要求的基本技能及享受相关服务时的满意度。[5]

21世纪初，越来越多的人认为，对全部人群和对个体患者的忽视都是不符合伦理的。这场争论主要论点在于环境的变化和资源的利用，而非低质量的医疗卫生保健。然而，这些环境问题都与"公地悲剧"①密切相关，在这一"悲剧"中，每当许多人使用一种共同的稀缺资源时，就会发生环境的退化（场景1.5）。鲁本认为：这就是医疗面临的实际情况[6]。如果每个临床医生和每个患者都越来越多地使用有限的医疗资源时，卫生资源总有一天会崩溃，而每个人也都会遭殃。

场景1.5　公地悲剧

情况：假如你是一个在公共土地上放羊的农民
按照习惯和传统，只允许你在公共土地上养20只羊，但你多养了一只，似乎没有人注意或介意。第二年你又多养了一只，第三年你又多养一只，以此类推。不幸的是，所有农民都采取了相同策略，直至到达临界点，然后整个生态系统崩溃，草不再生长，所有的羊都死了，这就是公地悲剧。

Apart from the danger of service breakdown, in healthcare it is also important to bear in mind that with increasing resource the balance between benefit and harm changes-with increasing resource investment benefit is subject to the law of diminishing returns whereas harm increases in direct proportion to the resources invested; indeed a point may be reached when the increased investment of resources will lead to a reduction in net benefit. Thus, it is important to be cautious about using increased resources, not simply from a financial perspective but also from the perspective of maximising the balance of benefit to harm for the population served.

During the 20th century, healthcare professionals provided health services on the assumption that 'more is better', however, there is a new paradigm for the 21st century:

In medicine there are three do's; the can do, the actually do and the should do. . . with the aging of the population and the proliferation of the can do, the increase in future healthcare capabilities and costs is an impending tragedy of the commons. The most important challenge for the 21st century is not to expand the can do; rather, it is to bring the care that is provided into line with the should do. Failure to do so will result in a healthcare system that will certainly be fiscally, if not morally, bankrupt. (6)

■ New skills for population medicine

This book, *How to Manage Population Medicine*, has been prepared to help both the general practitioner consortia involved in commissioning, and hospital and mental health specialists, both medical and nonmedical, to develop the knowledge and skills they need for the task of population medicine. It is focused primarily on the new responsibilities of clinicians, and in particular their responsibility to the whole population, not just their responsibility to the proportion of the population in contact with the service. For acute, unequivocal health needs, such as a broken leg, the whole population in need accesses the right service, but this is not the case for many people with chronic health problems.

The focus of management and leadership development in the last decade has been on managing an institution, a health centre or a hospital, although general practitioners have always had a focus on populations. The emphasis on quality improvement, on making care more effective and safer, work that is also focused on institutions, has been essential but is not sufficient to meet the challenges of the 21st century. Practising clinicians today should take responsibility for not just

除了卫生资源枯竭的危险，还需要意识到，在医疗卫生保健中随着投资的增加，损益平衡会发生变化：投资收益遵从收益递减规律，而投资风险则随着投资增多而增加。的确，当投资增多到达临界点后，增加资源投入所带来的净收益会逐渐减少。因此，谨慎使用已增加的资源非常重要，不仅要从财务角度，还要从为所服务的人群获取最大利益的角度来考虑。

在20世纪，医疗卫生专业人员是基于"越多越好"的理念来提供医疗卫生保健服务的，然而在21世纪，出现了新的范式：

> 医学有"三做"——能做、实做、该做。随着人口老龄化，以及"能做"的激增，未来医疗服务能力和成本的增加将是一个迫在眉睫的"公地悲剧"。21世纪最大的挑战不是扩充"能做"，而是我们所提供的照护应以"该做"为原则。如果做不到这一点，我们的医疗卫生保健服务体系一定会出现崩溃——不在财政上就在道德上。[6]

■ 群医学的新技能

《如何践行群医学》这本书将会帮助全科医生及医院、精神卫生专家掌握必要的知识和技能，以使他们（医学或非医学的）能够承担和开展群医学工作。这本书首要关注的是临床医生的新责任，特别是他们对整个人群的责任，而不仅是对那些已接触到医疗的人们负责。如前所述，对那些急性的、需求明确的疾病如腿部骨折，有医疗需求的人皆可以获得妥善处治，但这对许多有慢性疾病的患者来说，情况却不然。

在过去的十年中，尽管全科医生一直以人群为重点，但是管理和领导力开发的重点是管理机构，卫生中心或医院。强调质量改进，使医疗服务更有效、更安全，这些工作也是以机构为中心的，这至关重要但不足以应对21世纪的挑战。今天，临床医生实践中不仅应该对来专科就诊的患者负责，而且还应该对其需求可以直接或间接地通过专科服务的技能得到满足的人群负责。

the patients who happen to have made contact with the specialist service but also all the people whose needs could be met, directly or indirectly, by the skills of the specialist service. The skills for population medicine complement and supplement the skills that many clinicians have acquired during the last two decades. Although this new skill set includes general management skills and techniques to improve quality and safety, the skills that clinicians will need to maximise value for the whole population, as well as to improve quality and safety for individual patients, have not hitherto been covered. See Box 1.3.

Box 1.3 The skills for population medicine

- Maximising value
- Reducing waste and increasing sustainability
- Mitigating inequity
- Promoting health and preventing disease
- Creating systems
- Building networks
- Clarifying pathways
- Developing budgets
- Managing knowledge
- Engaging the population and patients
- Changing the culture

■ The need for medical leadership

Of all the skills needed to promote population medicine, that relating to changing the culture might be the most difficult to apply, but culture change is an integral part of leadership. Towards the end of the 20th century, it was accepted that a subset of clinicians had to be given training to develop management skills. Later on, the need to develop leadership skills was also recognised, based on the principle, long accepted in industry, that leadership and management although related required different skill sets: leaders are expected to shape and change culture, whereas managers work within it.

When we examine culture and leadership closely, we see that they are two sides of the same coin; neither can really be understood by itself. If one wishes to distinguish leadership from management or administration, one can argue that leadership creates and changes cultures, while management and administration act within a culture. (7)

群医学的新技能是对很多临床医生在过去20年获得的工作技能的补充和完善。尽管这套新技能包含了那些可以提高质量及安全性的一般的管理技能和技术。但是迄今为止，如何使医疗卫生保健对于全人群的价值最大化以及如何提高对个体患者的服务质量及安全性，临床医生依旧欠缺这些方面所需的技能。这就是群医学需要解决的问题（专栏1.3）。

专栏1.3 群医学的技能

- 价值最大化
- 减少资源浪费，提高可持续性
- 减少不平等
- 促进健康和预防疾病
- 构建体系
- 建立工作网络
- 理清工作路径
- 制订预算
- 知识管理
- 动员民众和患者
- 改变文化

■ 对医疗领导力的需求

在促进群医学所需的所有技能中，文化变革可能是最难得到应用的，但文化变革又是领导能力不可或缺的一部分。到20世纪末，大家普遍认同一部分临床医生需要接受培训以发展管理技能。此后，加上临床医生需要开发领导技能的观点也得到了认可。

当我们仔细研究文化和领导力时，我们会发现它们是一个硬币的两面；两者都不能真正地被单独理解。如果人们希望将领导力与管理或行政区分开来，可以认为领导力创造并改变了文化，而管理和行政则在文化中行事。[7]

Any new culture needs to be inculcated from the first day of professional education. Some medical schools have already recognised the need for a new curriculum to meet the demands and pressures of a world in which there are finite resources, as outlined by Cooke in the New England Journal of Medicine:

We must ensure that all students acquire a basic understanding of how medical care is financed, where national healthcare policies come from, and the politics that shape financing and workforce choices. (8)

This task of culture change will not be easy. Clinicians must continue to be committed to the individual patients in front of them, but in the decades to come they will also need to develop a commitment to the whole population, including to the patients they have never seen and may never see.

■ Questions for reflection or for use in teaching or network building

If using these questions in network building or teaching, put one of the questions to the group and ask them to work in pairs to reflect on the question for three minutes; try to get people who do not know one another to work together. When taking feedback, let each pair make only one point. In the interests of equity, start with the pair on the left-hand side of the room for responses to the first question, then go to the pair on the right-hand side of the room for responses to the second question.

- What are the ethical issues for clinicians whose only concern is for the patients who consult them?
- Although the introduction of free treatment under the NHS in 1948 freed many patients from anxiety about the costs of consulting, what was its effect on the power balance between doctor and patients?
- If we accept that responsibility for quality, equity and ensuring patients are treated with dignity are all essential aspects of good healthcare, are there any other responsibilities in addition to the six listed which clinicians need to fulfil in the 21st century?
- Why should all clinicians be explicitly responsible for these six dimensions or only a proportion of them?

要想使新文化扎根，就必须让学生在接受专业教育的第一天就沐浴在这种文化氛围中，反复熏陶。一些医学院校已经认识到需要设立一门新课程来应对在资源有限的世界里所面临的需求和压力。正如库克在《新英格兰医学杂志》上总结所言：

我们必须确保所有学生对医疗卫生保健的筹资方式、国家医疗政策的发展以及决定筹资和人力资源选择的方针政策有一个基本的了解。[8]

实现文化变革的目标绝非易事。临床医生必须致力于服务其面对的每位患者，同时也需要对所有需要帮助的人群做出承诺，包括那些他们尚未谋面甚至永远素昧平生的患者。

■ 互动思考题

如果在工作网络建设或教学中使用以下问题，可以将其中一个问题交给小组，让他们两人一组，思考3分钟，并尽量让彼此不认识的人一起工作。要求每组只能提出一个观点作为反馈。为了公平起见，让房间左侧的一组开始回答第1个问题，然后让房间右侧的一组开始回答第2个问题。

- 如果临床医生对只关注前来咨询就诊的患者，这将面临怎样的伦理问题？
- 尽管1948年在NHS下实行的免费治疗使许多患者摆脱了对咨询费用的焦虑，但它对医生和患者之间的权力平衡有什么影响？
- 如果我们忍痛确保医疗服务的质量、公平及患者在诊疗中得到尊重，这些职责都是好的医疗卫生实践的不可或缺的方面，那么除了本章提到的21世纪临床医生应当履行的6项职责外，还有哪些职责？
- 为什么所有的临床医生都应该明确地承担对本章提到的6项职责中的一部分或全部？

References

(1) Mitton, C. and Donaldson, C. (2004) Priority setting toolkit. A guide to the use of economics in healthcare decision making. BMJ Publishing Group (pp.5-6).

(2) Block, P. (1996) Stewardship: choosing service over self-interest. Barrett-Koehler.

(3) Holmgren, D. (2002) Permaculture. Holmgren Design Services (p.5).

(4) Goldberg, D. And Huxley, H. (1980) Mental Illness in the Community. The Pathway to Psychiatric Care. Tavistock Publications.

(5) Daniels, N. and Sabin, J.E. (2008) Setting Limits Fairly, Learning to Share Resources for Health. Oxford University Press (p.44).

———————————————————————————— 参 考 文 献 ———

（6）Reuben, D.（2010）Miracles, choices and justice; the tragedy of the future commons. JAMA 304; 467-468.

（7）Schein, E.H.（2004）Organizational Culture and Leadership. John Wiley & Sons Inc.（pp.10-11）.

（8）Cooke, M.（2010）Cost consciousness in Patient Care-what is Medical Education's responsibilities? NEJM 362; 1253-1254.

Chapter 2
MAXIMISING VALUE

第二章
价值最大化

This chapter will:

- distinguish between the two different types of meaning of value — the moral meaning and the economic meaning;
- give examples of the meaning of the term 'value' when it is used in an economic sene;
- distinguish between quality and value and describe their relationship;
- discuss ways in which the allocation of resources, either between programmes or within a programme, can increase value;
- discuss how the management of innovation and redundancy is essential to maximise value;
- define inappropriate and futile care and how variations in practice may indicate the presence of inappropriate care.

By the end of this chapter, you will have developed an understanding of:

- the difference between the economic meaning of the word value and the moral meaning;
- the relationship between quality improvement and value improvement;
- three types of lower value interventions;
- how those who allocate resources can maximise value, either by the process of allocation or by the way in which they handle innovation and disinvestment;
- how allocation decisions can be made not only between programmes but also within programmes, and even within the budget of resources available for a specific disease;
- the spectrum of care from necessary to futile;
- unwarranted variation and how this should be analysed;
- how variations in the level of health service activity, in particular high rates of intervention, may indicate inappropriate care and the need for patient decision aids.

■ The end of the quality era

For the last decade, the focus of healthcare managers and clinicians has been on quality improvement. However, as shown in Figure 2.1, focusing on quality alone improves, but does not maximise, value. Value is defined as doing the right things right to the right people.

本章涉及内容：

● 区分两种不同类型价值的含义——道德含义和经济含义；

● 举例说明"价值"一词在经济意义上的含义；

● 质量和价值两者之间的区别并描述两者之间的关系；

● 讨论项目之间或内部资源分配可以提升价值的不同方式；

● 讨论为什么管理创新和冗余对实现价值最大化至关重要；

● 定义何谓不当和无效医疗，以及实践中的差异如何说明存在不当医疗。

在本章末，读者将会深入理解：

● "价值"一词的经济含义与道德含义的区别；

● 质量提升与价值提升的关系；

● 3种低价值的干预措施；

● 负责配置资源的人员如何通过资源分配的过程，或者通过处理创新和减资的方式，以实现价值最大化；

● 不仅在项目之间，而且在项目内部，甚至在可用于特定疾病的预算范围内，如何做出资源配置的决策；

● 差异从必要到无效的照护排序；

● 不必要的差异以及如何分析；

● 医疗卫生服务活动水平的差异（特别是高干预率）是如何表明可能存在不当照护并需要患者辅助决策。

■ 质量时代的终结

在过去十年中，医疗卫生管理人员和临床医生一直致力于改善质量。如图2.1所示，仅注重质量可以提高价值，但不能使价值最大化。价值被定义为"为正确的人做正确的事"。

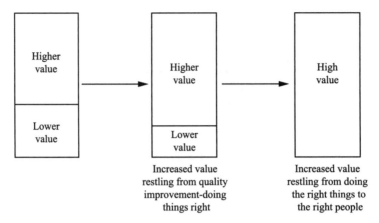

Figure 2.1 Doing the right things right to the right people

There is now a shift in emphasis from quality to value as signalled by an article entitled *The End of the Quality Improvement Movement: Long Live Improving Value* by Robert Brook, one of the most influential founders of the quality improvement movement.

Instead of trying to fill gaps in knowledge about the epidemiology of quality, the focus should be on developing an epidemiology of value, which contains both measurement of cost and quality, and is applicable to both the developed and the developing world. The results of this work would help to distinguish between a level of quality that is good value and the best available quality that may provide small improvements in health at enormous cost.(1)

As with any paradigm shift, the new paradigm of increasing value embraces and absorbs the older paradigm of improving quality. However, it is necessary to clarify the meaning of the term 'value' in this context.

■ The meanings of value

For an object, such as a book, it is possible to develop a definition stating what it is; however, for a concept, such as value, it is more productive to identify the various meanings of the term rather than a simple definition.

Value in any field must be defined around the customer, not the supplier.... Hence it is patient health results that matter, not the volume of services deliv-

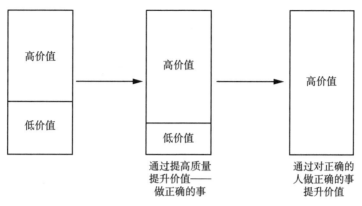

图2.1　对正确的人做正确的事

正如质量提升运动最有影响力的创始人之一罗伯特·布鲁克（Robert Brook）撰写的题为《质量提升运动的终结：提升价值万岁》的文章所表明的，现在的医疗卫生服务重点已从质量转向价值。

与其试图填补关于医疗卫生服务质量的"流行病学"认识上的空白，不如将重点放在建立与发展关于服务价值的"流行病学"上，它既包括成本的测量，也包括质量的测量，并且适用于发达国家和发展中国家。这项工作的成果将有助于区分具有良好价值的质量和需要花费巨大成本获得微小健康改善的最佳可及的质量。[1]

与任何范式转变一样，提升价值的新范式包含并吸收了提高质量的旧模式。然而，有必要澄清在此情形下"价值"一词的含义。

■ 价值的含义

对于书这样的物体而言，为其拟定一个定义说明其性质并非难事；然而，对于像价值这样的概念来说，识别该术语多重含义比单纯下定义更有成效。

任何领域中的价值必须围绕消费者而非供给者进行定义……因此，重要的是患者的健康，而不是提供的服务数量。然而，取得好的结果是有

ered. But results are achieved at some cost. Therefore, the proper objective is the value of health care delivery, or the patient health outcomes relative to the total cost (inputs) of attaining those outcomes. Efficiency, then, is subsumed in the concept of value. So are other objectives like safety, which is one aspect of outcome. (2)

There are many different meanings associated with the word 'value' when used in the context of healthcare.

The moral meaning: 'the status of a thing or the estimate in which it is held according to its real or supposed worth, usefulness, or importance' (a definition from late Middle English in the Shorter Oxford English Dictionary). This meaning of the word 'value', often used in the plural, is common in healthcare, for example, the hospital that states 'Our values are to promote patient choice', and 'We respect openness and honesty'. Another term to describe this meaning would be a 'principle'.

The economic meaning: one of the four variants of the term in the Shorter Oxford English Dictionary is 'that amount of some commodity, medium of exchange, etc. which is considered to be an equivalent for something else'; an example of the meaning from 1806 which is still relevant two centuries later is given as 'We could hardly be said to have value for our money' (3).

In healthcare, value is measured by the relationship between outcome and cost, as expressed by the following formula:

$$Value = Outcomes/Costs$$

However, because all healthcare can do harm as well as good, the formula needs to be amended to reflect this:

$$Value = (Good\ outcomes\text{-}bad\ outcomes)\ /Costs$$

As good and bad outcomes are determined by the decisions and actions of professionals, the value of a service depends on:

- *whether decision-making is evidence-based*;
- *the safety of the service*;
- *the quality of the service.*

成本的。因此，合适的目标应该是医疗卫生保健服务的价值或者患者的健康结局，应该与取得这些结局的总成本（投入）相适应。于是，价值的概念中包含效率。其他目标也是如此，比如安全，也是结果的一个方面。[2]

在医疗卫生保健领域中，"价值"一词有许多不同的含义。

道德含义："根据事情真实或应有的内涵、有用性或重要性而认为其应具备某个状态或估价。"（出自中世纪晚期《简明牛津英语词典》的英文定义）"价值观"这层含义多见于其英文名词的复数形式，在医疗卫生保健行业中很常见。例如，医院称"我们的价值观是优化患者的选择"，以及"我们尊崇开明守信的价值观"，而表达这个意思另外一个用词是"原则"。

经济含义：在《简明牛津英语词典》中，价值的4种含义之一是"某种商品的数量、交换的媒介（如货币、支票）等，可被认为与其他某种东西等价"。关于这个词，在1806年的一个用法的例子是"我们的钱花得值"，这个例子在两个世纪后仍然适用[3]。

在医疗卫生保健领域中，价值由结局和成本之间的关系来衡量，如公式所示：

$$价值＝结局/成本$$

由于任何医疗卫生保健都可能有利有弊，因此需要对公式进行修订如下：

$$价值＝（好结局－坏结局）/成本$$

专业人员的决策与行为决定了结局的好坏，而服务的价值取决于：

● 决策是否循证；

● 服务的安全性；

● 服务的质量。

Thus, the paradigms of high-quality healthcare, evidence-based decision-making and patient safety remain important, but the 21st century is the era of value in which the outcome is the dominant concern.

■ The meanings of outcome

Following the distinction of outcome from process by Avedis Donabedian, in the early literature on outcome, the most important step was to distinguish process measures from outcome measures. Process measures are easier to define and implement than outcome measures but have less validity. For example, a process measure would be the degree to which a hospital achieved certain safety standards; the outcome measure would be a hospital's standardised mortality ratio (SMR).

However, during the last decade, the focus has shifted to the patient's perception of outcome. Initially, it was thought that patient experience measured service quality with greater validity than patient satisfaction, which is greatly influenced by a patient's expectations. It is now clear that the patient's opinion of the outcome of care must be measured and not simply the patient's experience of the interpersonal aspects of care. Thus, patient-reported outcome measures (PROMs) are seen as outcome measures at least as important as the clinician's perception of the success of an intervention.

The patient's perception of outcome has also become important in the context of an increasing emphasis on the harm of healthcare. In the 20th century, the dominant preoccupation was the benefits of healthcare; in the 21st century, the dominant preoccupation will be the balance between benefit and harm, either from the perspective of the individual patient or from that of the population. In Matrix 2.1, the relationship between benefit and harm from an intervention for individual patients is shown.

		Benefits from Intervention (good outcome)	
		Present	Absent
Harm from Intervention (poor outcome)	Absent	Very good outcome	Disappointing for the patient: was the decision to intervent correct?
	Present	Parception of outcome dependant on the balance of good and harm and the patient's expectation when consenting (4)	Very bad outoome

Matrix2.1 Relationship of benefit to harm for individual patients

因此，尽管高质量医疗、循证决策和患者安全的行医范式仍然重要，但21世纪是一个以健康结局为主导的价值时代。

■ 结局的含义

在早期关于结局的文献中，阿维迪斯·多纳贝迪安指出结局和过程的区别，最重要的步骤是如何区分过程指标和结局指标。过程指标比结局指标更容易定义和实施，但有效度较低。例如，过程指标可以是医院达到某些安全标准的程度；而结局指标可以是医院的标准化死亡率（SMR）。

然而，在过去的十年里，患者对结局的看法越来越得到重视。最初，人们认为对于服务质量来说，患者体验的可信性高于患者满意度，因患者满意度受其期望的影响较大。现已明确的是，必须衡量患者对医疗卫生保健结局的看法和意见，且不只是患者接受了多少来自医务人员方面的关怀。因此，应把患者报告结局测量（patient-reported outcome measures，PROMs）与临床医生对干预成功的看法视为同等重要。

在日益强调医疗卫生保健伤害的背景下，患者对结局的感受也变得十分重要。在20世纪，人们想的都是医疗卫生保健带来的益处；而在21世纪，无论是患者个人还是公众，最主要的关注点都是利弊之间的平衡。矩阵2.1对个体患者实施干预的利弊关系。

		干预产生疗效（良好结局）	
		有	无
干预造成损害（不良结局）	无	良好结局	令患者失望：决定干预是否正确
	有	对结局的看法取决于利弊的平衡和患者同意干预时的期望[4]	极差结局

矩阵2.1 对个体患者实施干预的利弊关系

To ensure that a high proportion of patients have a good outcome, in addition to making sure that only interventions associated with strong evidence of doing more good than harm are delivered safely and at high quality, the clinician leading a service must take several different approaches:

- *To ensure that every patient facing a fateful decision makes it fully informed;*
- *To ensure that the culture of the clinical service is one in which inappropriate or futile care is discouraged.*

■ Lower-value healthcare

The fact that an intervention is effective, i.e. there is strong evidence that it does more good than harm, does not necessarily mean that it is of high value either to the population or to an individual. The value of an intervention depends on the context in which it is offered, which then determines whether its use is appropriate.

Assessments of the effectiveness of an intervention are objective, whereas assessments of the appropriateness of an intervention are subjective. Clinical judgement is used to place an intervention on the spectrum of appropriateness (see Figure 2.2).

NECESSARY	APPROPRIATE	NAPPROPRIATE	FUTILE

Figure 2.2 The spectrum of appropriateness

There are many definitions of all of the terms on the appropriateness spectrum. However, one of the definitions of a 'necessary' procedure is given in the quotation below:

We define a procedure as necessary-or crucial-if all four of the following criteria are met:

The procedure must be appropriate.

It would be improper care not to recommend this service.

There is a reasonable chance that the procedure will benefit the patient. Procedures with a low likelihood of benefit but few risks are not considered necessary.

The benefit to the patient is not small. Procedures that provide only minor benefits are not necessary.

为确保多数患者能获得良好结局，除了要向患者提供利大于弊的循证干预措施以保证安全、确保质量的方式外，临床医生还需采取一些不同的方法：

- 确保每个患者在面临重大决定时都能充分知情；
- 确保临床服务的文化是不鼓励采用不当或无效的医疗服务。

■ 低价值的医疗卫生保健

某种有效的干预措施（例如，有强有力的证据表明其利大于弊）不一定意味着它对群体或个体都有很高价值。干预的价值取决于提供干预的环境，而环境又决定了干预是否适当。

对干预有效性的评估是客观的，而对干预适当性的评估是主观的。临床判断被用于判别干预措施适当性的程度（图2.2）。

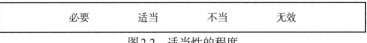

| 必要 | 适当 | 不当 | 无效 |

图2.2 适当性的程度

适当性程度里的所有术语都有许多定义，然而，"必要"流程的定义之一如以下引文所述：

若能同时满足以下4个标准，我们则将此流程定义为必要或关键的：

- 服务流程必须适当。
- 不推荐不适当的医疗服务。
- 该程序有很大可能性令患者受益。低风险低受益的程序则被认为是不必要的。
- 对患者的益处不应该小，只带来微小益处的流程被认为是不必要的。

In conclusion, necessity ratings can be used together with appropriateness ratings to address not only the overuse of procedures but also to indicate limited access to care through underuse of procedures. Key words: appropriateness; necessity; crucial; guideline panels. (5)

It is generally accepted that the definition of 'appropriate' in relation to a procedure is that outlined by Kahan et al:

...a procedure is termed appropriate if its benefits sufficiently outweigh its risks to make it worth performing, and it does at least as well as the next best available procedure. A procedure is termed inappropriate if the risks outweigh the benefits. (6)

Although it may be easy to agree upon the general definition of a term such as an 'appropriate' procedure, it is not as easy for a group of doctors to reach agreement when asked to identify whether an intervention is appropriate for a particular patient. Furthermore, it is not easy to reach an agreement on the definition of 'futility' when considered in relation to individual patients, as the following extract from one of the key books on futile intervention shows:

Schneiderman and Jecker have suggested that a treatment should be considered futile when it has not worked once in the last 100 times it was tried. Waisel and Truog attack this definition by noting that the criterion is statistically equivalent to saying that a therapy is futile if physicians are 95% confident that it would be successful no more than 3 in 100-a mathematical truism that Schneiderman et al. had themselves admitted in an earlier publication. (7)

Clinicians may disagree about what is or is not an appropriate procedure or what is or is not futile care for an individual, but they tend not to be aware that the care offered by their service would be considered inappropriate by other doctors or people in other professional groups.

Two different types of data can highlight the possibility of inappropriate care:

- *time trends — as the rate of operation increases, the probability of inappropriate care increases because treatment is offered to people who are less severely affected;*

总之，必要性评级和适当性评级可以一起使用，不仅可以解决医疗卫生服务的过度使用，还可以杜绝因服务使用不足而导致获得医疗卫生保健的机会有限。关键词：适当性、必要性、临界值、临床指南。[5]

卡汉等人对流程"适当"的定义如下：

……如果一项程序带来的益处远超过其风险，而且它至少应该与备选方案一样好，那么它是值得实施的，这个流程也是适当的。若其风险大于益处，则该流程是不适当的。[6]

虽然在诸如"适当"流程这类术语的一般定义上可能容易达成共识，但对于一些医生来说，一项干预对于特定患者来说是否合适就没那么容易达成一致意见了。此外，就患者个体而言，要就"无效"干预的定义达成一致并不容易。正如以下节选自一本关于无效干预的重要书籍的内容所示：

施耐德曼和杰克尔建议，如果一种疗法在过去100次尝试中没有一次奏效，就应该认为它是无效的。威塞尔和特鲁格反驳这个定义，指出该标准相当于在统计学上说，如果医生有95%的把握认为某项治疗成功的概率不超过3%，那么就认为该疗法是无效的——施耐德曼等人在自己早期发表的论著中承认了这一点，并且在数学上进行了证明。[7]

临床医生可能就某特定患者的医疗程序是否适当或治疗是否无效存在分歧，但他们往往意识不到，其他医生或专业团体也会认为他们所提供的医疗服务不当。

两种不同类型的数据可以体现不当医疗服务的可能性：

● 时间趋势——手术率增加，不当医疗服务的可能性亦随之增加，因为可能会出现过度治疗。

- *analysis of variation — high rates of intervention in a population, as revealed by the Dartmouth Atlas of Health Care (8) and The NHS Atlas of Variation in Healthcare (10), indicate the possibility of unwarranted variation.*

■ More is not necessarily better

Many elective operations are now performed much more frequently than they were in the past. For instance, the rate of cataract operations in England increased significantly from 1989 to 2004 (see Figure 2.3).

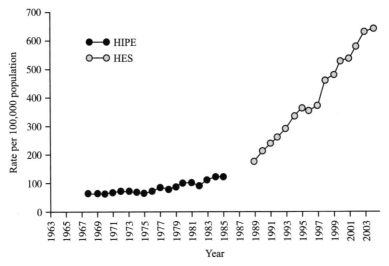

Figure 2.3 Rate of cataract operations per 100,000 population, 1989-2004 (reproduced from the British Journal of Ophthalmology, Tiarnan Keenan, Paul Rosen, David Yeates, Michael Goldacre, Volume 91, pages 901-904©with permission from *BMJ* Publishing Group Ltd) [Goldacrefig, Atlas 1.0]

Initially, an increase in the number of operations performed represents addressing what everyone would agree was unmet need, such that the increase in the volume of interventions provided is deemed necessary. However, with time, as the absolute number of operations and the rate of intervention increase, people whose need is less severe receive the intervention, and it is debatable whether the care can be classified as 'necessary'.

Avedis Donabedian was the first to describe what happens as the volume of medical care provided to a population increases and the threshold for intervention changes, originally published in Explorations In Quality Assessment & Monitoring (10), but latterly in Introduction to Quality Assurance in Health Care (11). He

● 差异分析——如达特茅斯卫生保健地图集[8]和NHS卫生保健差异地图集[10]显示的那样，人群干预率高表明有不合理差异的可能性。

■ 并不是越多越好

如今，许多非必需的手术比过去开展得更多了。例如从1989—2004年，英国的白内障手术率就显著上升（图2.3）。

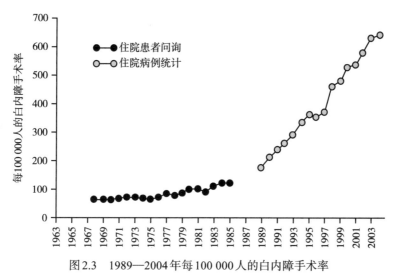

图2.3　1989—2004年每100 000人的白内障手术率

（引自 *British Journal of Ophthalmology*，Tiarnan Keenan，Paul Rosen，David Yeates，Michael Goldacre，BMJ，91卷，901-904，经BMJ许可）

起初，手术量的增加解决了每个人未满足的需求，因此，增加干预措施成为了必然之事。然而随着时间推移，增加的手术量和干预率导致需求并非那么强烈的人也会得到干预，在这种情况下所提供的医疗服务是否"必要"则有待商榷。

阿维迪斯·多纳贝迪安首次说明了为人群提供的医疗服务增加并将更多人纳入干预范围会造成什么结果。他的研究最初发表在 *Explorations in Quality Assessment & Monitoring* 中[10]，后期又发表在 *Introduction to Quality Assurance in Health care* 上[11]。他指出，随着资源投入的增加：每增加一个

pointed out that as the amount of resources invested increases, the benefit that results from each unit of increase becomes smaller, known as the law of diminishing returns, whereas the amount of harm done increases in direct proportion to the investment of resources (see Figure 2.4).

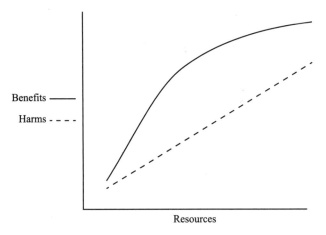

Figure 2.4 The Law of Undiminished Harm

Thus, there is a point when the investment of additional resources will lead to reduction in net benefit or health gain calculated by subtracting the harm from the benefit, as shown in Figure 2.5. The turning point beyond which additional resources do not result in any increase in value Donabedian called the point of optimality.

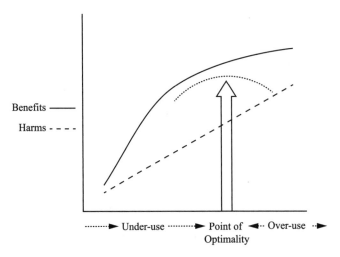

Figure 2.5 The relationship between resources, benefit and harm——under-use, optimality and over-use

单位所产生的效益会变小，这就是收益递减规律；所造成的损害与资源的投入成正比（图2.4）。

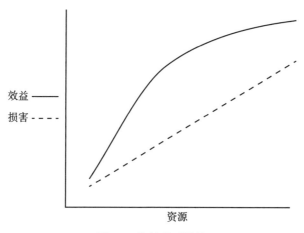

图2.4　收益递减规律

因此，到了一定程度，额外的资源投入将导致净效益或健康收益的减少，其计算方法是从获益中减去损害，如图2.5所示。超过这个转折点，额外的资源投入不会带来任何的价值增加，多纳贝迪安称之为最优点。

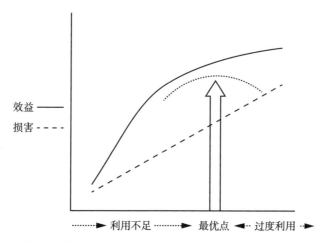

图2.5　资源、获益和损害之间的关系——利用不足、优化和过度利用

Clinicians need to be aware of the point at which the balance between benefit and harm becomes unfavourable. Donabedian described the task as:

The balancing of improvements in health against the cost of such improvements. The definition implies there is a 'best' or 'optimum relationship' between costs and benefits of health care, a point below which more benefits could be obtained at costs that are low relative to benefits and above which additional benefits are obtained at costs too large relative to corresponding benefits. (11)

■ Unknowing and unwarranted variation in practice

The groundbreaking research of Professor John Wennberg at Dartmouth Medical School demonstrated that there were large and unknown variations in clinical practice, such as in the rate of knee operations. Furthermore, much of this variation was not only unknown but also unwarranted, which he defined as:

Variation in the utilization of health care services that cannot be explained by variation in patient illness or patient preferences. (12)

It is important to appreciate that clinicians responsible for providing a greater level of intensity of care were convinced that the level of care was appropriate. No conscientious clinician provides inappropriate care consciously. Every clinician believes that what they deliver is appropriate but, because most clinicians and most local services work in isolation, there is very little awareness of what others do. For this reason, the clinician intervening twice as often as the mean and the clinician intervening half as often as the mean believe they are intervening at the 'right' rate, as does the clinician who intervenes at the mean rate. None of them should necessarily be confident about the level of intervention including the clinician intervening at the mean rate because that may also encompass many inappropriate interventions.

The identification of inappropriate practice can be achieved in several different ways:

- *by encouraging clinicians to visit other services or 'buddy' with another service so that exchanges can be arranged-working in another service can be illuminating;*

临床医生需要意识到利弊平衡开始变得不利时的临界点。多纳贝迪安将此描述为：

健康改善与其改善所需成本之间的平衡点。这个定义意味着，在医疗卫生保健的成本和收益之间存在着"最优"或"最佳关系"，低于该临界点，可以以相对于收益而言较低的成本获得更多的收益；高于该点，则说明需要以相对于收益而言过高的成本方能获得额外收益。[11]

■ 临床实践中的未知和不合理的差异

达特茅斯医学院约翰·温伯格教授的一项开创性研究表明，在临床实践中存在着巨大且未知的差异，例如膝关节手术率。此外，此类差异大多数不仅是未知的，而且是不合理的，他将其定义为：

卫生服务利用的差异，不能用患者病情或患者偏好来解释。[12]

负责上一级医疗服务的临床医生，确信他们所提供的服务水平是合适的，意识到这点非常重要。尽责的临床医生绝不会故意提供不当的医疗服务。尽管每个临床医生都认为其提供的医疗服务是适当的，但因为许多临床医生和当地机构是独立工作的，所以他们并不了解其他人的做法。因此，采取的干预强度是均值的两倍或一半的临床医生们都会认为自己是以"正确"的强度进行了干预。他们中的任何人都不能确信其干预水平（包括以平均比率进行干预的临床医生）是正确的，因为这也可能包括许多不当干预。

不当干预的鉴别可以通过以下几种途径实现：

● 鼓励临床医生走访其他机构或兄弟单位，以便开展交流——了解不同机构可能会带来启发；

- *through peer review of cases and case-notes*;
- *by identifying and investigating variation in activity——the possibility that there is over-use or under-use of a service is raised if rates of activity are higher or lower than in comparable services caring for similar populations.*

The appropriateness of an intervention is distinct from its effectiveness. Appropriateness is determined by the values of the patient. Therefore, it is essential that the patient's values are incorporated into any clinical decision about whether or how to intervene. This can be done by promoting shared decision-making via the use of patient decision aids.

Variations analysis and shared decision-making are both ways in which the 'right' outcomes can be achieved for populations and individual patients, respectively. Furthermore, these methods are inter-related. When rates of intervention are high, the balance of benefit to harm may be beyond the point of optimality from a population perspective. From the perspective of an individual patient, the types of outcome that have to be considered are also different because, as Wennberg highlighted, when there are more resources:

- *less severely affected people are being offered interventions*;
- *for each person, the magnitude of benefit that can be expected is reduced because their problem is less severe to start with, however, the likelihood and magnitude of harm experienced is the same as for more severely affected people.*

Wennberg states that if an operation is performed on a patient who does not understand the risks they face, and who would not have accepted the offer of the operation if they had been so informed, the service has operated on 'the wrong patient'.

■ Seven steps to increase value

Although steps to improve quality and safety lead to better outcomes, there are further steps that a clinician responsible for delivering healthcare to a population can take to increase value in addition to these two core functions of service management (see Box 2.1)

● 开展病例和病历记录的同行评议；

● 识别和研究卫生服务的差异——如果某项干预强度高于或低于针对人群的可比干预强度，则干预过度或干预不足的可能性就会增加。

如前所述，干预的适当性不同于其有效性。适当性由患者的价值观决定。因此，将患者的价值观融入临床决策（是否或如何干预）中是至关重要的。可以通过应用患者辅助决策工具来促进共同决策。

差异分析和共同决策两种方法都可以使得患者群体和个体获得"正确"结果。此外，这些方法是相互关联的。当干预率很高时，从群体的角度来看，利弊平衡可能会超过最优点；从个体的角度来看，需要考虑的结局也是有所不同的，因为正如温伯格强调的，当资源更多时：

● 病情较轻者也会得到干预；

● 对每个人而言，由于其问题从一开始就不太严重，所以预期获益减少，但其受到伤害的可能性和程度与病情更重的人却相差无几。

温伯格指出，如果对不了解手术风险的患者进行了手术，而当其充分知情后可能选择不接受手术，那么这个手术对象就是"错误的患者"。

■ 提升价值的7个步骤

虽然改善质量和安全性会带来更好的结果，但除了以上两个服务管理的核心功能外，负责人群健康的临床医生还可以采取进一步的措施来提升价值（专栏2.1）。

Box 2.1 Seven steps to increase value in healthcare

- Negotiating well with payers and commissioners
- Allocating resources to different patient groups to achieve optimality
- Within each group of patients with the same condition, allocating resources to achieve the optimal balance of prevention, diagnosis, treatment and care
- Ensuring the right patients are seen by the service
- Encouraging innovation and disinvestment to increase value
- Getting the right outcome for the right patient
- Reducing waste (see Chapter 3)

Negotiating well with payers and commissioners

Those who pay for, or commission, healthcare allocate resources to different programme budgets. The allocation of resources in NHS England across 23 programme budget categories is shown in Table 2.1.

Table 2.1 Programme budgeting estimated England-level gross expenditure for programmes in 2010/2011[1]

Programme budgeting category code	Programme budgeting category	Gross expenditure 2010/11 (£ billion)
1	Infectious Diseases	1.80
2	Cancers & Tumours	5.81
3	Disorders of the Blood	1.36
4	Endocrine, Nutritional and Metabolic Problems	3.00
5	Mental Health Disorders	11.91
6	Problems of Learning Disability	2.90
7	Neurological	4.30
8	Problems of Vision	2.14
9	Problems of Hearing	0.45
10	Problems of Circulation	7.72
11	Problems of the Respiratory System	4.43
12	Dental Problems	3.31
13	Problems of the Gastro-Intestinal System	4.43
14	Problems of the Skin	2.13

---

[1] http://www.dh.gov.uk/health/2012/08/programme-budgeting-data/

专栏2.1 提升医疗卫生保健价值的7个步骤

- 付费者和委托人进行良好的沟通。
- 将资源分配给不同的患者群体，以达到最优效果。
- 在每一组病情相同的患者中，分配资源以达到预防、诊断、治疗和保健的最佳平衡。
- 确保那些真正有需求的患者得到服务。
- 鼓励创新并减少投入以提升价值。
- 让正确的患者能够得到正确的健康结局。
- 减少浪费（见第三章）。

与付费者和委托人进行良好的沟通

那些支付或委托医疗卫生保健服务的人负责将资源分配给不同项目预算。NHS在23类项目预算上的资源分配情况见表2.1。

表2.1 2010/2011年度英国医疗服务项目的预算[①]

项目预算类别编号	项目预算类别	2010/2011年度总支出（亿英镑）
1	感染性疾病	18.0
2	癌症和肿瘤	58.1
3	血液疾病	13.6
4	内分泌、营养和代谢疾病	30.0
5	精神健康障碍	119.1
6	学习障碍	29.0
7	神经系统疾病	43.0
8	视力障碍	21.4
9	听力障碍	4.5
10	循环系统疾病	77.2
11	呼吸系统疾病	44.3
12	口腔疾病	33.1
13	消化系统疾病	44.3
14	皮肤病	21.3

① http://www.dh.gov.uk/health/2012/08/programme-budgeting-data/

（续表）

Programme budgeting category code	Programme budgeting category	Gross expenditure 2010/11（£billion）
15	Problems of the Musculo-Skeletal System	5.06
16	Problems due to Trauma and Injuries	3.75
17	Problems of the Genito-Urinary System	4.78
18	Maternity and Reproductive Health	3.44
19	Conditions of Neonates	1.05
20	Adverse Effects and Poisoning	0.96
21	Healthy Individuals	2.15
22	Social Care Needs	4.18
23	Other Areas of Spend/Conditions	25.95
Total		107.00

One of the key responsibilities for the clinician managing a service is to try to gain additional resources from the organisation that allocates money to all programmes of care. In an era of constraint, this responsibility may become one of trying to prevent the service from suffering cuts.

In times of growth, clinicians managing services have become accustomed to bid for resources to add to the programme budget for their service, relying on the institution allocating resources among programmes to fund in their favour based on the case of need submitted. The case of need, or business case, has traditionally been based on evidence of effectiveness and cost-effectiveness.

Let us take the situation among three programme budgets-respiratory disease, gastro-intestinal disease and cancer-as an example. The respiratory services programme has bid for additional resources. If successful, the respiratory services programme would receive an increased amount of resources and thereby a greater proportion of the budget, whereas the services for people with gastro-intestinal disease and cancer would retain the same absolute amount of resources but receive a smaller proportion of the budget. When making decisions about resource allocation among different programmes of care, decision-makers have to take as a starting position the inherited levels of resource allocation（see Figure 2.6）.

（续表）

项目预算类别编号	项目预算类别	2010/2011 年度总支出（亿英镑）
15	肌肉－骨骼系统疾病	50.6
16	外伤和创伤疾病	37.5
17	生殖泌尿系统疾病	47.8
18	产妇和生殖健康	34.4
19	新生儿健康	10.5
20	不良反应和中毒	9.6
21	个体健康	21.5
22	社会关怀需求	41.8
23	其他领域的支出/问题	259.5
合计		1070.0

临床医生在服务管理中的关键职责之一是设法从那些为所有医疗服务项目拨款的机构中获得额外资源。在一个资源稀缺的时代，这种职责可能会是尽量防止医疗项目开支被削减。

在经济增长时期，管理服务的临床医生已经习惯于竞标资源以增加其服务的方案预算。机构会根据提交的需求为他们偏爱的项目分配资源。需求案例或项目企划通常是根据有效性和成本效益的证据来决定的。

以呼吸系统疾病、消化道疾病和癌症3个项目预算为例。针对呼吸系统的医疗服务项目已竞标获得了额外资源。顺利的话，呼吸系统医疗服务项目将获得更多的资源，从而在财政预算中占更大的比例；而为胃肠道疾病和癌症患者提供的医疗服务的绝对数量可能不会变化，但在预算中所占的比例可能会减少。当决策者在不同的医疗服务项目之间分配资源时，需要以此前承继的资源配置水平作为出发点（图2.6）。

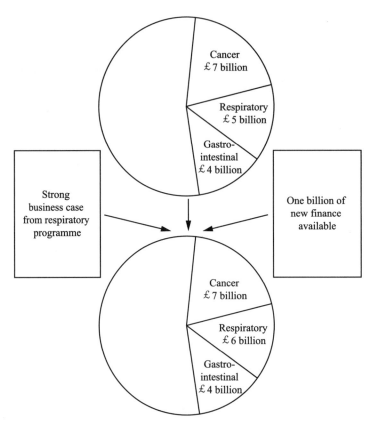

Figure 2.6 Winning resources for the respiratory programme budget when resources are increasing

In times of fiscal constraint when there is no growth in resources, payers and commissioners have to switch resources from one programme budget to another, using a process called marginal analysis.

The task of measuring costs and benefits should be done through marginal analysis. This involves starting with a particular mix of services and analysing changes in that mix. If resources can be shifted to produce greater benefit then this should be done.(13)

The aim is to achieve Pareto optimality, that is, the point at which allocative efficiency is at its maximum when the distribution of resources is such that shifting a pound from one budget to any other would produce no more value. Needless to say, this state of Pareto optimality, analogous to a state of divine grace, has never been reached in any health service. It should be noted that the allocation of resources across programme budget categories in NHS England (Table 2.1) did not necessarily result from a process of logical analysis. It simply represents the end result of decades of ad-hoc decisionmaking.

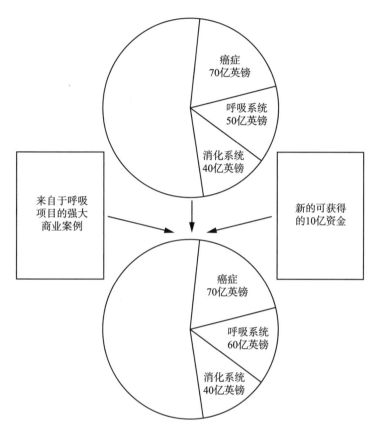

图2.6 当资源增加的情况下，为呼吸系统的服务项目争取更多预算

　　在财政紧张时，资源总量难以增长，医疗支付方与委托方需要将资源从一个项目调整到另一个项目，所依据的是边际分析法。

　　衡成本和效益的任务应该通过边际分析来完成。这涉及从特定的服务组合开始，并分析组合中的变化。如果资源可以通过项目间的转移产生更大的效益，那么就应该对资源进行转移。[13]

　　该方法的目标是实现"帕累托最优"。所谓的帕累托最优可以理解为：当从一项预算中转移一英磅到其他任何预算中将不会产生更多价值时，配置效率已达到最大。毋庸赘言，帕累托最优类似于神的恩赐，在任何医疗服务中都未曾实现过。需要注意的是，NHS跨项目预算类别的资源分配（表2.1），不一定是逻辑分析过程的结果，只代表几十年临时决策的最终结果。

In future, the clinician responsible for delivering a service to one subgroup of the population will have to prepare a bid or business case in which it is argued that:

- *there is no waste or lower-value activity in their budget*;
- *if resources were switched from another programme budget, the population as a whole would receive better value (Figure 2.7)*.

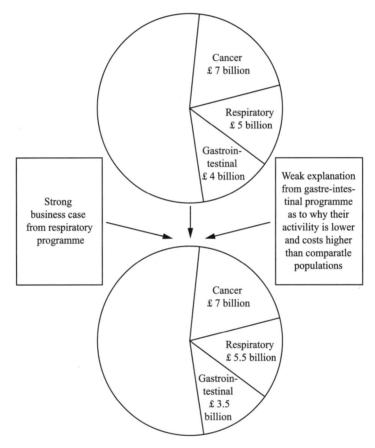

Figure 2.7 Winning resources for the respiratory programme budget when there is no growth in resources

However, before starting marginal analysis, payers and commissioners will expect clinicians to examine their own budgets. Payers and commissioners will want assurance that:

未来，负责向某一人群提供服务的临床医生必须准备一份投标书或商业企划，其中需要说明以下几点：

● 他们的预算中没有浪费或低价值的活动；
● 如果从另一个项目预算中调拨资源，整个人群将获得更好的价值（图 2.7）。

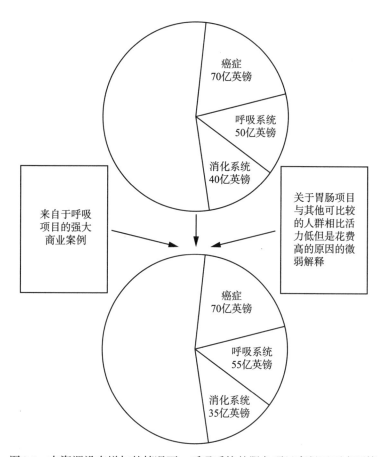

图2.7　在资源没有增加的情况下，呼吸系统的服务项目赢得了更多预算

然而，在进行边际分析之前，那些医疗卫生费用的支付方和委托人期望临床医生审视他们的预算，并保证以下内容：

- *the entire programme budget is allocated optimally to the different conditions within that programme;*
- *after allocation the service achieves high value from the resource allocation.*

Allocating resources to different patient groups optimally unless general practitioners have a special interest in a particular condition or aspect of medicine, as generalists they need to distribute their resources among all their patients as best they can, given that as generalists they deal with all types of health problem. Specialists, however, are frequently faced with more explicit decisions about the allocation of resources among a small number of patient groups or sub-specialties, although specialists also have to take account of patients with rare diseases.

When there are increases in health service investment, the clinician who is a manager bids for more resources to increase the amount invested in the condition for which increased need has been identified-in a sleep apnoea service, for example, where need has increased due to improved diagnosis and the development of new technology. However, when there is no increase in health-service investment, the most likely source of additional finance for sleep apnoea will be from within the respiratory diseases programme budget (see Figure 2.8), which in England is about £100 million per million population.

It is rare that the decision-maker is able to make a decision completely rationally. They must use what Herbert Simon called 'bounded rationality', a principle that the main proponents of systems thinking have adapted and promoted.

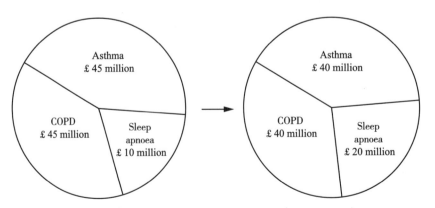

Figure 2.8 Finding resources for sleep apnoea from within the respiratory programme budget (figures are approximations)

- 整个项目预算在该项目内的不同条件下得到最优分配；
- 在分配后，可通过资源再分配实现服务的高价值。

全科医生需要处理各种类型的健康问题，除非他们对某一疾病或医学某一方面有特殊兴趣，否则他们需要尽可能地把资源分配给所有患者。与全科医生不同的是，专科医生最常面临的问题是如何在少数的几组患者之间或亚专科之间分配资源，有时还需要考虑罕见病患者群体。

当医疗卫生保健投资增加时，作为管理者的临床医生会为已确定需要增加需求的服务内容竞标，以争取更多的资源。例如，诊断技术的改进和新技术的发展导致睡眠呼吸暂停综合征的相关服务需求增加时，医生就可以寻求增加这方面的资源。但是，当医疗卫生保健投资没有增加时，睡眠呼吸暂停综合征的额外资金将最可能来自呼吸系统疾病的项目预算（图2.8），在英格兰，这一预算约为每百万人口1亿英镑。

决策者很少能够完全理性地做出决定。他们必须使用赫伯特·西蒙所称的"有限理性"（bounded rationality），这是系统思维倡导者已经习惯遵循并提倡的原则。

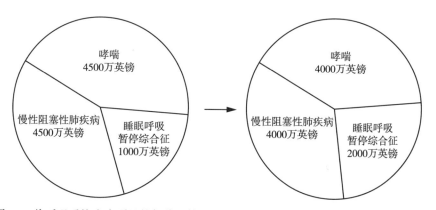

图2.8　将呼吸系统疾病项目的部分预算调整用于睡眠呼吸暂停综合征（数字为近似值）

Bounded rationality arises because human cognitive capabilities, as wonderful as they are, are overwhelmed by the complexity of the systems we are called upon to manage. Chapter 1 discussed bounded rationality; here I repeat Herbert Simon's (Administrative Behaviour, 1957, p.198) principle of bounded rationality: 'The capacity of the human mind for formulating and solving complex problems is very small compared with the size of the problems whose solution is required for objectively rational behaviour in the real world —— or even for a reasonable approximation to such objective rationality'. (14)

In making decisions about the care for a population, such as the population of London or a subgroup of the population with common needs such as people with respiratory disease, three factors have to be taken into consideration (see Figure 2.9):

- *Evidence of good and bad effects of all the interventions;*
- *The value the population places on the benefits and harms of each care option;*
- *The other needs of the population.*

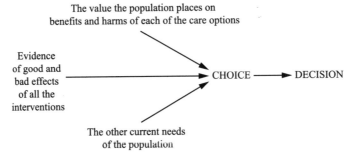

Figure 2.9 Relating the evidence to the needs and values of the population

As the evidence is rarely 100% conclusive and it is impossible to model precisely the impact of the resources used on the whole population, the decision-maker will have to make a value judgement. However, judgement is a subtle concept that has more than one meaning. Furthermore, value judgements often have important ethical elements. Thus, judgement is exercised not only in weighing the different options but also in understanding, calculating and managing the ethical elements of the decision, a complexity that has been described by Herbert Simon.

有限理性的产生是因为尽管人类的认知能力很强大，但也会受困于人们需要管理的系统的复杂性。本书第一章讨论了有限理性，在此，我重复赫伯特·西蒙（《管理行为》，1957，第198页）对于有限理性原则的描述："与所需要解决的问题的规模相比，人类大脑梳理和解决复杂问题的能力非常小，现实中客观理性的行为或者是近似这种客观理性的行为需要这些问题的解决方案。"[14]

在对某人群（如伦敦的人群）或有共同需求的某个人群亚组（如呼吸系统疾病患者）进行医疗服务决策时，必须考虑3个因素（图2.9）：

- 所有干预措施所产生影响（正面、负面）的证据；
- 人群对每种医疗服务选择的利弊所持有的价值观念；
- 人群的其他需要。

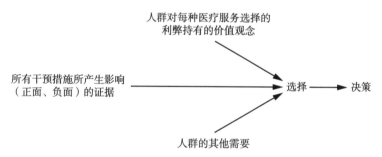

图2.9　将证据和人群的需要及价值取向联系起来

由于证据几乎不能百分百确定，加之不可能精确地估计出所使用资源对整个人群的影响，因此决策者必须对价值做出判断。然而，判断是一个微妙的概念，有不止一种含义。此外，价值判断往往具有重要的伦理要素。因此，判断不仅要权衡不同选择，还需要理解、计算、管理决策的伦理要素。赫伯特·西蒙曾描述过这种复杂性。

- *It is here that judgement enters. In making administrative decisions it is continually necessary to choose factual premises whose truth or falsehood is not definitely known and cannot be determined with certainty with the information and time available for reaching that decision...*
- *In ordinary speech there is often confusion between the element of judgement in decision and the ethical element. This confusion is enhanced by the fact that the further the means-end chain is followed, i.e. the greater the ethical argument, the more doubtful are the steps in the chain, and the greater is the element of judgement involved in determining what means will contribute to what ends.*(15)

This exercise of judgement can bring the clinician responsible for the budget into conflict with colleagues, particularly if those colleagues do not feel any responsibility towards the stewardship of resources. In this situation, it can be helpful to provide colleagues with examples of types of activity that can be classified as being of lower value to populations and patients (see Box 2.2).

Box 2.2 Interventions or services of lower value

- There is clear evidence of ineffectiveness of evidence that they do more harm than good
- There is no or weak evidence of effectiveness but the intervention/service is not being delivered in a context that would enable the collection of evidence to judge effectiveness, e.g. not being delivered as part of an ethically approved, welldesigned research project-these interventions are often referred to as 'innovations' or 'developments'
- There is evidence of effectiveness, but the intervention/service is being offered to patients whose characteristics are different from those of the patients in the original research studies that produced the evidence of effectiveness
- They consume resources that would produce more value, i.e. a better balance of benefit to harm, if invested in another intervention/service for the same group of patients

Achieving optimal balance between prevention, diagnosis, treatment and care for a single group of patients

Value-based decisions also have to be made when considering a single group of patients-people with chronic obstructive pulmonary disease (COPD), for example. The decision to switch resources from domiciliary oxygen to triple therapy could be regarded as one that can be based on evidence of effectiveness because it concerns the best mix of therapies for patients at a particular stage in the course of their disease. However, decision-making about care for a group of patients can include a value judgement because:

● 这就需要判断了：在行政决策中，需要不断对事实前提进行选择；但我们无法判断这些事实前提的真伪，也无法根据现有信息、在有限的时间内判断其确切性。

● 在日常对话中，我们常会混淆决策判断因素和伦理因素。这种混淆因为以下事实而加剧：如果遵循方法－目的链，也就是说，道德争论越激烈，在通过方法实现目的的推导链条上的因素就越可疑，在决定采用何种手段以利于实现何种目的时所需考虑的判断因素也就越多。[15]

这种判断会使负责预算的临床医生与同事发生冲突，特别是当这些同事对资源管理不承担任何责任时。在这种情况下，向同事举例说明那些对人群和患者价值较低的活动类型可能会有助于他们对情况的理解（专栏2.2）。

专栏2.2 价值较低的干预或医疗服务

● 有明显的证据表明这些干预措施并无效果或弊大于利。
● 没有或有较弱的证据证明干预的有效性，且干预或医疗服务没有在可以判断其有效性的情景下实施，如没有以经过伦理审批和良好实验设计的科研项目的一部分的形式提供给患者，这种干预或医疗服务往往被称为"创新项目"或"在发展中的项目"。
● 证据表明其有效，但被提供干预/医疗服务的患者与原始研究中证明有效的患者对象人群特征不同。
● 如果对同一组患者施以另一种干预/照护，资源使用会产生更高的价值，即能在利弊间得到更好的平衡。

在同一病种患者之间实现预防、诊断、治疗和照护最佳平衡

当考虑同一病种患者群体时（例如慢性阻塞性肺疾病患者），也需要基于价值的决策。将资源从家庭氧疗转换为三联疗法的决策可以被视为是一个基于有效性证据的决定，因为它涉及患者在疾病发展过程中特定阶段的最佳疗法组合。但是，对同一病种患者的医疗卫生保健服务决策可能会包括价值方面的判断，其原因是：

- *the options are rarely directly comparable;*
- *each option may be championed by a colleague who is an enthusiast for their particular intervention, ready to argue why they need more resources or why they should be spared a cut.*

This process of achieving an optimal balance in resource allocation for a single group of patients is referred to as 'within-system marginal analysis'. In this type of marginal analysis, the options have to be considered within the limits of the finite resources available for that particular health problem. For instance, the clinician in charge of respiratory services for a population who has already allocated all the resources optimally to the three principal conditions-asthma, sleep apnoea and chronic obstructive pulmonary disease (COPD) -may have to use judgement to decide on the balance of resources between treatment and rehabilitation.

Consider the options facing the clinician responsible for a comprehensive COPD service. They can allocate resources to five different types of intervention — prevention, diagnosis, treatment, rehabilitation and end-of-life or palliative care (see Figure 2.10).

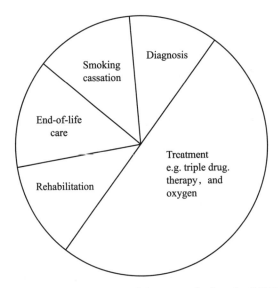

Figure 2.10 Components of the system budget for COPD

To support clinicians in the allocation of resources within a service, tools have been developed by a team at the London School of Economics (LSE) that can

- 这些选项几乎不具有直接的可比性；
- 每一种选择都可能被特定干预措施的狂热者所倡导，他们随时准备为争取更多资源或避免被削减的缘由而争论不休。

为某同一病种患者取得资源分配的最佳平衡的过程可被称为"系统内边际分析"。在这种边际分析中，必须在针对特定健康问题的有限资源范围内考虑各种选择。例如，对于已经将所有资源以最优方式分配给3种主要疾病：哮喘、睡眠呼吸暂停综合征和慢性阻塞性肺疾病的人群时，负责呼吸系统医疗卫生保健的临床医生可能不得不判断治疗和康复之间的资源平衡。

当临床医生提供慢性阻塞性肺疾病综合医疗卫生保健时，可能会遇到不同的选择，他们可以将资源分配到5种不同类型的干预：预防、诊断、治疗、康复和临终或姑息治疗（图2.10）。

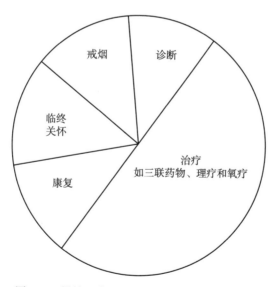

图2.10 慢性阻塞性肺疾病系统预算的组成部分

为了支持临床医生在服务中对资源的分配，伦敦政治经济学院（LSE）

enable the value of different choices to be estimated and displayed in order to stimulate discussion and debate. ①

- *This tool was used by healthcare professionals to assess the relative value of different interventions for COPD. They concluded that: the current sequence of management may need reordering so that interventions such as stop smoking and consideration for referral to pulmonary rehabilitation should happen before any trial of triple therapy.* (16)

The decision to switch resources from treatment to prevention, or vice versa, is a value judgement encompassing ethical elements, as is the decision to switch resources from asthma to COPD or from respiratory disease to cancer.

Ensuring the right patients are seen

In Chapter 1, it was emphasised that one of the most important actions in population medicine is to ensure that a specialist service sees the right patients, and that the patients being supported by generalists receive the right care. This requires the clinician practising population medicine to be concerned about all the people in the population who have a particular condition, and to support all the clinicians working with that population irrespective of whether those clinicians are generalists or specialists.

Taking a population approach to health services is likely to reduce inequity because there is usually a higher proportion of people from disadvantaged and deprived communities in the subgroup of the population who are either not seen by the specialist service or who do not receive a particular intervention.

Encouraging innovation and disinvestment to maximise value

Another way of classifying the value judgements that a clinician responsible for delivering services to a population has to make is to consider them as investment or disinvestment decisions. Decisions about investment or disinvestment are generated by the desire to fund an innovation created by either another organisation, such as a new drug or a new piece of equipment, or someone who works in or uses the service (see Figure 2.11).

---

① http://www.health.org.uk/news-and-events/newsletter/star-combining-valuefor-money-with-patient-involvement/

的团队开发了一些工具，可以估算和展示不同选择的价值，从而促进讨论和辩论。①

- 这一工具用来都助医疗工作者评估针对慢性阻塞性肺疾病不同干预的相对价值。他们的结论是：目前慢性阻塞性肺疾病的管理顺序可能需要重新排序，以便在任何三联疗法试验之前，应先采取如停止吸烟和考虑肺部康复转诊的干预措施。[16]

将资源从治疗转向预防，就像决定将资源从哮喘转向慢性阻塞性肺疾病或从呼吸道疾病转投向癌症（反之亦然），是一个包含各种伦理因素在内的价值判断。

确保那些适宜的患者得到服务

第一章强调了群医学最重要的行动之一是确保专科医生能够看到适宜的患者，并确保接受全科服务的患者能得到适宜的医疗救治。这要求从事群医学的临床医生关注人群中患有特定疾病的所有患者并支持治疗这些患者的全部临床医生，无论他们是全科医生还是专科医生。

群医学践行很可能可以减少不公平，因为在弱势人群和贫困社区的亚人群中往往有较高比例的居民既没有得到专科医疗服务也没有得到特殊干预。

鼓励创新并减少投入以实现价值最大化

另一种给价值判断的分类方法是，当践行群医学的临床医生作决策时，必须将价值判断视为投资或撤资的决定。有关投资或撤资的决定建立在想要投资另一机构（如新药或新设备）或另一人（使用该服务或为其工作）的创新项目渴求之上（图2.11）。

---

① http://www.health.org.uk/news-and-events/newsletter/starcombining-valuefor -money-with-patient-involvement/

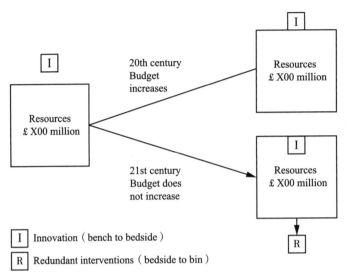

Figure 2.11 The funding of innovation from disinvestment

Encouraging higher-value and discouraging lower-value innovation

Innovation is usually associated with starting new services or procedures. However, two other activities are of greater importance if innovation is to be managed well:

- *stopping starting — that is, stopping the drift into practice of lowervalue interventions;*
- *starting stopping — that is, stopping lower-value activities so that resources may be released for re-use, referred to as disinvestment.*

Those who manage clinical services have to be alert to the arrival of new technology that does not increase value or, if it does, is introduced before other interventions deemed to be of lower value have been stopped or scaled down. Controlling procurement and the order book allows new technology to be appraised, but new technology can bypass appraisal processes in various ways:

- *through being lent by the developer;*
- *by masquerading as research;*
- *by being given by the manufacturer without an initial charge;*
- *or bought by a charity in an attempt to change clinical practice and force the hand of the budget-holder.*

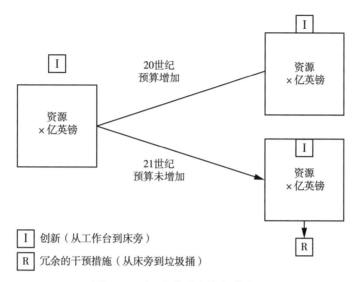

I 创新（从工作台到床旁）

R 冗余的干预措施（从床旁到垃圾桶）

图2.11 减少投资为创新提供资金

鼓励高价值创新，避免低价值创新

创新通常与启动新服务或新程序有关；但要管理好创新，另外两项活动更为重要：

- 停止启动（stopping starting）——阻止低价值干预措施付诸实践；
- 启动停止（starting stopping）——停止低价值的活动以便资源可以被释放而另作他用，也被称为撤资。

临床服务管理者要谨慎使用不能增加价值的新技术，如果新技术能够增加价值，应在低价值干预措施被叫停或缩减之后引入。通过管控采购和订单，可以对新技术进行评估。但是，新技术能以各种方式绕过评估过程：

- 通过开发者租借给其他人；
- 伪装成研究项目；
- 在改变临床实践的尝试中，由制造商免费提供；
- 或者由慈善机构收购，试图改变临床实践，并左右预算持有者的决定。

Those who manage clinical services must also be alert to the arrival of new knowledge that can increase value. In an ideal world, all clinicians would be motivated not only to adopt new technology but also to monitor new knowledge in order to identify evidence of higher-value interventions, or evidence of ineffective or lower-value interventions which would lead them to start stopping a service or a long-standing clinical practice. However, people tend to be slow to adopt new knowledge even that which does not increase costs——for instance, the evidence that a checklist used before an operation reduces the risk of harm (17). Clinicians may not start stopping long-established practices unless they are motivated to find the resources to fund an innovation that they want and which they believe will add value to the service.

In England, NICE has made a major contribution to improving the management of innovation by the NHS, particularly where new drugs are concerned. New equipment and new procedures, such as new surgical operations or new models of service delivery such as a new screening programme, are more difficult to manage:

- *the research to assess their effectiveness is more difficult to undertake*;
- *implementation is much more difficult, being dependent on the skill of the surgeon or the functioning of a multidisciplinary team, or both.*

These difficulties surrounding the management of surgical innovation were addressed in a workshop organised by the Nuffield Department of Surgery, Oxford. This discussion led to a series of articles published in *The Lancet*. The first of the articles described a new paradigm for evaluation of surgical innovation (see Box 2.3).

Box 2.3 A five-stage paradigm for the development of innovative surgical practices (18)

1. Innovation
2. Development
3. Early dispersion and exploration
4. Assessment
5. Long-term implementation and monitoring

In the final article in *The Lancet* series, it was emphasised that the evaluation of new surgical interventions had more in common with the evaluation of complex interventions than it did with pharmacological interventions. This observation led to the proposal of a set of recommendations for the management of surgical innovation (19).

临床服务管理者也必须对能够增加价值的新知识保持敏感性。在理想情况下，所有的临床医生不仅会主动采用新的技术，而且也会主动获取有关高价值的、无价值或低价值的干预措施证据的新知识。这些证据会引导临床医生停止某项服务或长期临床实践。即使是像"手术前使用检查表可以降低伤害风险"[17]这类不会增加成本的知识，人们接受的速度仍然缓慢。临床医生可能不会叫停长期临床实践惯例，除非有动力鼓励他们去寻找资源进行他们想要的且相信会增加服务价值的创新。

英国国家卫生与临床优化研究所（NICE）为改善NHS的创新管理做出了重大贡献，尤其是在涉及新药的领域。新设备和新程序（如新外科术式）或提供服务的新模式（例如新的筛查方案）更难以管理，是因为：

- 开展效果评估的研究难度较大；
- 实施起来要困难得多，这要依赖于外科医生的技能或多学科团队的合作或两者兼而有之。

在牛津大学纳菲尔德外科系组织的一次研讨会上，围绕手术创新管理的这些困难得到了解决。这次讨论促成了一系列文章在《柳叶刀》上发表。其中第一篇文章描述了评价外科创新的新范式（专栏2.3）。

专栏2.3 发展外科手术创新实践的五阶段范式[18]

1. 创新
2. 发展
3. 早期应用
4. 评估
5. 长期应用和监测

《柳叶刀》系列的最后一篇文章强调了新手术干预的评估与复杂干预评估相比的共同点比与药理干预评估相比的共同点更多。这一观察结果导致了一系列外科创新管理建议的提出[19]。

When compared with the management of innovation, it is more difficult to manage the drift to inappropriate and futile care. The phenomenon of drift has been described by David Eddy (20) as being three battles to watch in the 1990s. He highlighted that one of the main factors increasing healthcare costs was 'changes in the volume and intensity' of clinical practice. He argued that this apparently inexorable increase in the volume and intensity of clinical practice must be managed if increasingly scarce resources are to be used effectively.

When an evidence-based innovation is first introduced, it is provided to a group of patients who have characteristics similar to the characteristics of the patients in the original research study in which the evidence base was generated. However, clinicians often have to use their judgement because in clinical practice there are very few patients completely identical to the patients in the original research study. This is because the study design often stipulates entry criteria that are rarely encountered in clinical practice. For instance, the entry criteria for a heart-failure trial might be restricted to people with heart failure under 65 years of age with no co-morbidities, whereas most patients with heart failure are over 65 years of age and have other conditions or co-morbidities. Thus, although clinicians may give the intervention to a tightly defined group of patients to begin with, over the years the intervention may be offered to other patients who have different indications or co-morbidities or who may be less severely affected.

Encouraging disinvestment from lower-value interventions

For the person managing a department or clinical service, there are several approaches to promoting disinvestment in lower-value interventions:

- *encouraging innovation within a fixed budget, safe in the knowledge that clinicians will have to do less lower-value work;*
- *encouraging disinvestment directly, which requires a framework clinicians can use to identify lower-value activities (see Box 2.4).*

To maximise value, it is essential to manage both innovation and disinvestment; leaving the maximisation of value to natural evolution is a high-risk strategy unlikely to succeed.

与创新管理相比，更难以改变的是扭转不当或无用的医疗卫生保健措施。这一"漂移"现象被大卫·埃迪认为是20世纪90年代3个值得关注的挑战之一[20]。他强调，医疗卫生保健成本增加的主要因素之一是临床实践中"数量和强度的变化"。他认为，如果要有效利用日益稀缺的资源，要加强管理在数量和强度上明显不断增加的临床实践。

当首次引入一项循证创新时，它被提供给一组特征与生成证据库的原始研究中患者特征相似的患者。然而，由于很少有患者与原始研究中的患者完全相同，临床医生在日常临床实践中往往不得不自行判断。这是因为在原始研究设计中通常规定的纳入标准在临床实践中很少遇到。例如，心力衰竭试验的纳入标准可能局限于65岁以下没有任何合并症的心力衰竭患者，而大多数心力衰竭患者是65岁以上有合并症的患者。因此，虽然临床医生一开始可能只对一组严格定义的患者进行干预，但多年以后，可能会对其他有不同适应证、合并症或症状较轻的患者进行干预。

鼓励从低价值干预中撤资

对于临床或部门管理者来说，有几种方法可减少对低价值干预措施的投入：

- 鼓励在固定预算范围内进行创新，确保临床医生尽量减少低价值工作；
- 鼓励直接撤资，这需要一个评估工具，临床医生可以使用它来识别那些低价值的活动（专栏2.4）。

要实现价值最大化，必须同时管理创新并减少投资。将价值最大化留待于自然选择实现，是一种不太可能成功的高风险策略。

Box 2.4 Framework to identify lower-value activities

- As specialists, are we seeing patients who could be managed equally as well by general practitioners?
- Are there clinical activities for which there is no evidence of benefit that we could stop?
- Are there clinical activities for which there is no supporting evidence that we could stop or have a trial to investigate stopping?
- Can we identify waste, i.e. non-clinical activity that adds no value? (See Chapter 3.)

Getting the right outcome for each individual patient

Changing the traditional view of the 'right' patient outcome

For decades, the definition of 'right' was established by medical opinion until Archie Cochrane published his book Effectiveness and Efficiency in 1972 (21). The application of Cochrane's principles to clinical practice was first called 'clinical epidemiology' (22) in a publication of that title written by the team from McMaster University, where so much of the leading work in knowledge management in medicine has been done. From the work at McMaster University, the concept of evidence-based medicine has been developed (18), which emphasises that the making of clinical decisions should be based on best current evidence and not established medical opinion.

Evidence-based medicine (EBM) requires the integration of the best research evidence with our clinical expertise and our patient's unique values and circumstances. (23)

Personalising decisions

The 'right' thing for individual patients is determined by the decisions made by clinicians and patients. For every million population, many decisions are made in the 40,000 consultations that take place daily. These decisions may be shared between clinicians and patients to a greater or lesser degree during a consultation, but many are taken by either clinicians or patients outside the consultation, such as a patient's decision not to take the medication prescribed for them. The total number of decisions daily is difficult to estimate, but it could be more than 200,000 per million population. These decisions influence both patient outcomes and cost.

Although the development of evidence-based decision-making, supported by services such as NHS Choices and NHS Evidence, has increased the probability of a good outcome, evidence is only one factor in the clinical decision, as illustrated

专栏2.4 用于识别低价值活动的框架

- 作为专科医生，我们所诊治的患者是否也可以在全科医生那里得到同等的治疗？
- 我们是否可以停止那些缺乏有益证据的临床活动？
- 对于没有得到证据支持的临床活动，我们是否可以停止或开展试验以使之停止？
- 我们能否识别浪费（如没有附加值）的非临床活动（见第三章）？

使每一位患者都能得到正确的医疗结局

改变有关"正确"患者结局的传统观点。

数十年来，"正确"的定义建立于医学观念之上，直至1972年阿奇·科克伦出版其著作《效果和效率》*Effectiveness and Efficiency*[21]。科克伦的理论在临床实践应用中第一次被称为"临床流行病学"[22]是在麦克马斯特大学的团队撰写的一份出版物中的标题里，该大学在医学知识管理方面做了大量的领先工作。从麦克马斯特大学的工作中，循证医学的概念得到了发展[18]，它强调临床决策应该基于当前最好的证据，而不是既定的医学观点。

循证医学（evidence-based medicine，EBM）要求把最佳研究证据、临床专家意见、患者个人价值观和具体情况整合在一起。[23]

个性化决策

对患者个体做出的"正确"诊疗是由临床医生和患者共同决定的。对每百万人口来说，每天进行的40 000次医疗询诊中会产生许多决策。这些决策或多或少在就诊时由临床医生和患者共同做出；但也有不少是由临床医生或患者本人在诊疗过程之外决定的，例如患者决定不服用为其开具的处方药物。每天的医疗决策总数很难估计，但是在每百万人口中可能会超过200 000次决策。这些决策对患者的医疗结果和费用都产生影响。

虽然在英国国家医疗服务体系选择（NHS Choices）和英国国家医疗服务体系证据（NHS Evidence）等服务的支持下，循证决策的发展提高了良好结

by the simple model of a treatment decision shown in Figure 2.12. From the patient's perspective, the need is for the right intervention, namely, an intervention for which there is a high probability of benefit and a low probability of harm, taking into account the unique clinical condition and values of the patient.

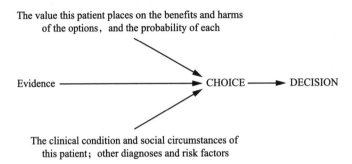

Figure 2.12 Relating the evidence to the needs and values of a particular patient

In the paradigm of evidence-based medicine, the use of best current evidence in decision-making is emphasised, but the clinician needs to relate the evidence, which has often been produced during research studies on patients who are different from the type of patient seen in clinical practice, to the unique clinical needs of each patient. This task can be referred to as personalised medicine.

...two key questions that are most frequently asked by clinicians about applying the results of randomised controlled trials and systematic reviews to decisions about their individual patients. Is the evidence relevant to my clinical practice? How can I judge whether the probability of benefit from treatment in my current patient is likely to differ substantially from the average probability of benefit reported in the relevant trial or systematic review? (24)

In addition, the development of our understanding of the human genome raises the possibility of using genetic tests to determine which particular treatment option would be best for a particular patient, an activity referred to as pharmacogenomics or precision medicine.

We define precision medicine as the provision of care for diseases that can be precisely diagnosed, whose causes are understood, and which consequently can be treated with rules-based therapies that are predictably effective.

Another term 'personalized medicine' is often used for this phenomenon that we're calling 'precision medicine'. (25)

局的概率，但正如图2.12治疗决策的简单模型所示，证据仅是临床决策中的因素之一。就特定临床状况利患者个体自身价值观而言，从患者的角度来看，需要的是正确的干预，即考虑到患者独特的临床条件和价值观，采取一种获益概率高、伤害概率低的干预。

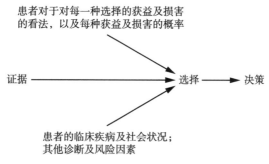

图2.12　患者需求和价值观与医疗证据的关联

在循证医学的范式中强调将当前的最佳证据用于制订决策。但这些证据常来源于那些与临床实际患者情况有差异的科学研究。临床医生需要将这些证据与每个患者实际医疗需求相结合，即所谓"个体化医疗"（personalized medicine）。

……临床医生最常问的两个关键问题是：如何将随机对照试验和系统综述的结果应用于对患者个体的决策。证据是否与我的临床实践相关？我如何判断目前的患者从治疗中获益的概率是否可能与相关试验或系统性综述中报告的平均获益概率有显著差异？[24]

此外，随着我们对人类基因组研究的逐步深入，根据基因检测判定对特定患者效果最佳治疗方案的可能性也相应得到了提高，这被称为"药物基因组学"（pharmacogenomics）或"精准医疗"（precision medicine）。

我们将精准医疗定义为"对于能够准确诊断疾病及其病因，因此，可通过基于规范的、具有可预测效果的疗法进行治疗的疾病所提供的医疗照护"。

另一个术语"个性化医疗"经常被用于"精准医疗"的情况。[25]

Preference-sensitive decisions

The third factor in any decision is the patient's values, that is, what value the patient places on the nature of the good and bad outcomes and on the probabilities of each outcome occurring. In some clinical situations, the issues are clear, such as in the choice of treatment for fractured neck of femur, but in others, such as in the treatment of prostate cancer, the different options for intervention have different consequences. To help patients make the decision best for them, it is essential they are given:

- *complete information about the probabilities of good and bad outcomes*;
- *the opportunity to reflect on how these relate to their values*.

The man considering different treatment options for prostate cancer needs support to reflect on whether it is more important for him to avoid incontinence or impotence. Even when the consequences of intervention are less dramatic, in knee replacement for example, the patient needs to reflect on the degree of knee pain and stiffness they are currently experiencing and to consider the possibility that the operation may not be completely successful or could make the pain and stiffness worse. This type of decision has been called a preference-sensitive treatment decision.

Preference sensitive treatment decisions involve making value trade-offs between benefits and harms that should depend on informed patient choice. (26)

In a report for the King's Fund, Mulley et al. have called for an end to the 'silent mis-diagnosis' of patients (27), defined as the failure to diagnose the patient's preferences even though the clinician has diagnosed the disease accurately.

The need for patient decision aids

No fateful decision should be made in avoidable ignorance. (28)

There is now a range of resources to improve decision-making, both for patients and clinicians, many of which were developed by Foundation for Informed Medical Decision Making. The term given to the most structured of these decision-making tools is the patient decision aid.

偏好敏感决策

在任何决策中的第三因素是患者的价值观，即患者个人对结局好坏及其发生概率所持的态度。在某些临床状况下，问题很容易解决，如股骨颈骨折的治疗选择；但在其他情况下，如治疗前列腺癌时，选择不同治疗方案会带来不同的结局。因此，为帮助患者做出最佳决策，给予以下信息至关重要：

- 关于好坏发生概率的完整信息；
- 患者有机会考虑这些与个人价值观之间的关系。

男性患者在选择前列腺癌治疗方案时，需要得到支持来考虑避免尿失禁或性功能障碍哪一个对于自身来说更为重要。当治疗效果并不显著时，这一原则也需要得到贯彻，如膝关节置换术要考虑患者当前膝关节疼痛及僵硬的程度，还需考虑到该手术可能并非百分百成功，甚至加剧疼痛僵硬的程度等。此类决策被称为偏好敏感决策。

偏好敏感决策包括利与弊之间的权衡，应该由患者在知情的情况下做出选择。[26]

在英国国王基金的一篇报告中，穆勒等人呼吁终结对患者"沉默的误诊"[27]，沉默的误诊是指：即使在疾病诊断准确的情况下，临床医生仍未能了解患者个人在治疗选择上的倾向。

患者决策辅助工具（patient decision aids）的必要性

应该避免在信息匮乏下做出重大决策。[28]

当前有一系列资源都可以用来改善患者及临床医生的决策制定，其中很多都是由医疗知证决策基金会（Foundation of Informed Medicine Decision Making）提供的。在这些决策工具中，最结构化的一种被称为"患者决策辅助工具"。

Patient decision aids are designed to support patients in this process; they are intended to supplement rather than replace patient-practitioner interaction. They may be leaflets, interactive media, or video or audio types. Patients may use them to prepare for talking with a clinician, or a clinician may provide them at the time of the visit to facilitate decision making. At a minimum, patient decision aids provide information about the options and their associated relevant outcomes.(29)

To support patients and clinicians during shared decision-making, patient decision aids have been developed in recognition of the constraints that time places on face-to-face consultations. The consultation remains crucial because clinical judgement has an important part to play in identifying the patient's preferred style of decision making; many patients still want their clinician to make the decision. However, the consultation can be supplemented and complemented by decision aids.

There is now an extensive and strong evidence base about the problems patients face in making the choice that is right for them, and a growing evidence base about the steps that can be taken to improve a patient's decision-making (see Box 2.5). The steps to improve decision-making need to be managed as actively as the processes involved in the management of safety by the clinician responsible for a service.

Box 2.5 Steps that can be taken to improve decision-making (30)

- Presenting evidence about benefit or harm in relative terms rather than absolute terms results in the patients, and doctors, choosing different options; the use of absolute numbers, such as the number needed to treat (NNT), is more easily understood than presenting them in relative terms, such as relative risk. Recognising that the research literature has a positive bias thereby giving the impression of greater benefit than is the case
- Offering all patient full information about the options because it is not possible to predict how much information a patient will want on the basis of their age or educational attainment giving full information in a way that suits the needs of individual patients will not increase the demand for resources; indeed, evidence shows that it can decrease demand (27)
- Identifying patients' preferences for style of decision-making-not all patients like the same style: some prefer to take the lead, some prefer the clinician to take the lead, and some prefer shared decision-making (31)
- Improving clinicians' skills in identifying the patient's preferred style of decision-making many clinicians cannot discern which style of decision-making an individual patient prefers
- Using patient decision aids to help the patient weigh up the values they place on the benefits and the harms, and the probabilities of each outcome and to overcome the constraints of time in face-to-face decision-making

设计患者决策辅助工具是为了在决策过程中支持患者，他们的目的是补充而非取代患者与医生的互动。它们的类型可能是传单、交互式媒体、视频或音频。患者可以使用患者决策辅助工具为与临床医生的交谈做准备，临床医生也可以在就诊时提供患者决策辅助工具以方便决策。至少，患者决策辅助工具提供了关于选项及其相关结局的信息。[29]

为了在医患共同决策过程中给予更好的支持，也由于意识到医患面对面诊疗时的时间有限，人们开发了患者决策辅助工具。即使有了患者决策辅助工具，医患之间的面对面诊疗仍至关重要；因为临床判断在确定患者偏好的决策方式中非常重要，多数患者仍希望由临床医生为自己做出决策，而决策辅助工具可由面对面诊疗进行补充和完善。

当下已有广泛有力的实证基础，让患者在面临问题时做出适合自己的选择；也有了越来越多的证据来改善患者决策的步骤（专栏2.5）。改进决策的步骤需和安全管理相关过程一样，需要由负责医疗的医生进行积极管控。

专栏2.5　可用于改善决策的步骤[30]

- 呈现结果损益证据时，以相对术语而不是绝对术语来提供有关获益或伤害的证据，会导致患者和医生做出不同的选择；用绝对术语如"需治疗人数（number needed to treat，NNT）"比用相对专术语如"相对风险（relative risk，RR）"，更易于被人们理解。要注意研究文献往往有正向偏倚，其显示的获益可能会优于实际情况。这一点十分重要。
- 因为无法通过患者年龄或受教育程度来预测其对信息的需求量，所以向所有患者提供可选方案的完整信息。提供能满足患者需求的完整信息并不会花费更多资源；事实上，有证据表明这反而可以降低需求[27]。
- 识别患者的决策偏好风格。患者的偏好风格各不相同：某些患者偏好由自己主导，某些偏好由临床医生主导，还有些则偏好共同决策[31]。
- 提高临床医生识别患者决策偏好风格的技能：许多临床医生并不能辨别某患者在决策时的偏好风格。
- 用患者决策辅助工具来帮助患者权衡损益。患者决策辅助工具也会凸显每一种结果的概率，以克服医患面对面诊疗时决策时间不足的限制。

However, it is clear that many fateful decisions are still made in 'avoidable ignorance'. Some of these fateful decisions concern elective surgery, others are about cancer treatment, and many are about end of life care. Indeed, the importance of distinguishing effectiveness and quality from outcome is particularly pertinent during end-of-life care. Many people receive effective, high-quality interventions when the outcome they most desire is a good death in their own home. It is not possible to maximise value for a service and for a population without maximising the value for each individual patient.

■ Questions for reflection or for use in teaching or network building

If using these questions in network building or teaching, put one of the questions to the group and ask them to work in pairs to reflct on the question for three minutes; try to get people who do not know one another to work together.When taking feedback, let each pair make only one point, In the interests of equity, start with the pair on the left-hand side of the room for responses to the first question, then go to the pair on the right-handside of the room for responses to the second question.

- What is the best way to explain value to members of the public meeting to consider the budget of a health service?
- When looking for greater value, should the focus be on marginal analysis or on the main budget for a programme?
- How can clinicians be best encouraged to disinvest?
- In what way can patient decision aids help an individual patient make the decision that is right for them?
- What are the responsibilities for the clinician when ensuring that patients make the decision that is right for them?
- What steps could be taken to reduce inappropriate and futile care?

References

(1) Brook, R.H. (2010) The End of the Quality Improvement Movement: Long Live Improving Value. JAMA, 304: 1832.

(2) Porter M.E. (2008) What is Value in Health Care?Harvard Business School. Institute for Strategy and Competitiveness. White Paper.

(3) Gray, J.A.M. (2007) Better Value Healthcare. Offox Press.

(4) Gigerenzer, G. and Edwards, A. (2003) Simple tools for understanding risks from innumeracy to insight. Brit. Med.J. 327: 741-744.

然而，许多决策仍然是在"可规避的无知"情况下做出的。某些重大决策涉及择期手术，有些则包括癌症治疗，还有很多涉及临终关怀。事实上，区分疗效和质量与结果对临终关怀尤为重要。许多临终患者虽然接受了有效且高质量的干预，但他们最希望的往往是在自己家中平静离世。脱离了患者个人价值的最大化，服务和群体价值的最大化也就无从谈起了。

■ 互动思考题

如果在工作网络建设或教学中使用以下问题，可以将其中一个问题交给小组，让他们两人一组，思考3分钟，并尽量让彼此不认识的人一起工作。要求每组只能提出一个观点作为反馈。为了公平起见，让房间左侧的一组开始回答第1个问题，然后让房间右侧的一组开始回答第2个问题。

- 向审议医疗卫生预算的公众会议的成员解释价值的最佳方式是什么？

- 在寻找更大价值时，重点应放在边际分析上还是放在方案的主要预算上？

- 如何最好地鼓励临床医生撤资？

- 患者决策辅助工具在哪些方面可帮助每个患者制定正确决策？

- 为确保患者决策正确，临床医生的职责是什么？

- 可以采取哪些步骤来减少不当和无效医疗？

参 考 文 献

(5) Gray, J.A.M. (2005) The Resourceful Patient. Offox Press.

(6) Kahan, J.P. et al. (1994) Measuring the necessity of medical procedures. Med. Care 32: 352-365.

(7) Schneiderman, L.J. and Jecker, N.S. (1995) Wrong Medicine: Doctors, patients and futile treatments. Baltimore: Johns Hopkins University Press.

(8) Dartmouth Atlas.

(9) Right Care (2010) The NHS Atlas of Variation in Healthcare. Reducing unwarranted

variation to increase value and improve quality. NHS. http: //www.rightcare.nhs.uk/ atlas/

(10) Donabedian, A.( )

(11) Donabedian, A.(2002) An Introduction to Quality Assurance in Health Care. Oxford University Press.

(12) Wennberg, J.E.(2010) Tracking Medicine. Oxford University Press.

(13) Mitton, C. and Donaldson, C.(2004) Priority setting toolkit. A guide to the use of economics in healthcare decision making. BMJ Publishing Group.(p.18)

(14) Sterman, J.D.(2000) In: Business Dynamics: Systems Thinking and Modeling for a Complex World. The McGraw-Hill companies Inc. p.598.

(15) Simon, H.A.(1997) Administrative Behaviour. A study of decision-making processes in administrative organizations.(Fourth edition). The Free Press.(p.60).

(16) Gray, J.A.M. and El Turabi, A.(2012) Optimising the Value of Interventions for Populations. British Medical Journal doi 10.1136/bmje6192.

(17) Gawande, A.(2003) Complications: A Surgeon's Notes on an Imperfect Science. Profile Books Ltd.

(18) Barkum, J.S. et al.(2009) Evaluation and stages of surgical innovation. Surgical Innovation and Evaluation, 1. Lancet 374: 1089-1096.

(19) McCulloch, P.A. and Schuller, F.(2010) Innovation or regulation?The IDEAL opportunity for consensus. Lancet 376: 1034-1035.

(20) Eddy, D.M.(1993) Three battles to watch in the 1990s. JAMA 270: 520-526.

（21）Cochrane, A. (1972) Effectiveness and Efficiency.

（22）Haynes, R.B., Sackett, D.L., Guyatt, G.H. and Tugwell, P. (2004) Clinical Epidemiology: How to Do Clinical Practice Research. Third edition. Lippincott Williams and Wilkins.

（23）Straus, S.E., Richardson, W.S., Glasziou, P. and Haynes, R.B. (2005) Evidence-Based Medicine. How to practice and teach EBM. (3rd Edition). Elsevier Churchill Livingstone (p.1).

（24）Rothwell, P.M. (2007) The Lancet. Treating Individuals: from randomised trials to personalised medicine. Oxford: Elsevier Limited.

（25）Christensen, C.M., Grossman, J.H. and Hwang, J. (2009) The Innovator's Prescription. A Disruptive Solution for Health Care. McGraw-Hill Professional.

（26）Christensen, C.M. (2003) The Innovator's Dilemma. Harper Business Essentials.

（27）Mulley, A., Trimble, C. and Elwyn, G. (2012) Patients' Preferences Matter: Stop the Silent Misdiagnosis. King's Fund, London.

（28）Mulley, A., personal communication.

（29）Elwyn, G. (2006) Developing a quality criteria framework for patient decision aids; online international Delphi Consensus process. BMJ, 333: 17-427.

（30）O' Connor, A.M. et al. (2007) Toward the 'Tipping Point': Decision aids and informed patient choice. Health Affairs 26: 716-725.

（31）Gigerenzer, G. and Gray, J.A.M. (2010) Better Doctors, Better Patients, Better Decisions. MIT Press.

Chapter 3
REDUCING WASTE AND INCREASING SUSTAINABILITY

第三章
减少资源浪费，提高可持续性

This chapter will:

- discuss the principal steps that can be taken to reduce the cost of healthcare;
- explain *muda* and its relevance to healthcare;
- provide a classification of different types of waste in healthcare;
- give a definition of sustainability;
- summarise the carbon reduction policy and plan for the NHS;
- outline the contribution of clinical practice to the carbon footprint of the NHS;
- summarise the key characteristics of low-carbon clinical practice.

By the end of the chapter, you will have developed an understanding of:

- the three steps that can be taken in health services to reduce cost;
- the Toyota seven-step approach to the reduction of waste, and how it has been adapted for healthcare;
- the meaning of cost-effectiveness analysis;
- the meaning of the term 'sustainable development';
- the way in which clinical teams can be motivated to take action on sustainability within a health service;
- the strategy that needs to be adopted to reduce the carbon footprint of clinical practice.

■ Responsibility for reducing waste and increasing sustainability

As discussed in Chapter 2, value is determined by the relationship between outcome and the resources used. It is the responsibility of the clinician serving a particular population to minimise the amount of resources used. Minimising resource use contributes to increasing sustainability. In the context of sustainability, the use of the term resources does not refer to money alone.

The relationship between reducing waste and increasing sustainability is shown in Figure 3.1. The reduction of waste in health services has immediate benefits because it can release resources which are then available to treat more members of the population. However, there are other longer-term benefits that result not only from reducing waste in healthcare but also from increasing the level of sustainability.

To be a good steward of resources for the population, clinicians practising population medicine need to reduce waste and increase sustainability, and not simply to cut budgets. Clinicians must prevent the waste of time, the time of both clinicians and patients, and the unnecessary use of carbon.

本章涉及内容：

- 讨论减少医疗花费的主要步骤；

- 解释浪费及其对医疗的重要性；

- 提出医疗浪费的不同分类；

- 给出可持续的定义；

- 汇总碳减排政策及其NHS的计划；

- 概括临床实践对NHS规划碳排放政策的贡献；

- 汇总低碳临床实践的主要特征。

在本章末，读者将会深入理解：

- 减少医疗成本的3个步骤；

- 丰田减少浪费的7步方法及其在医疗卫生服务中的应用；

- 成本－效益分析的含义；

- 可持续发展的含义；

- 激励临床团队在医疗服务实践中探索可持续发展的方法；

- 减少临床实践碳排放的策略。

■ 减少浪费和提高可持续性的责任

　　如第二章讨论的，价值取决于结果和所用资源之间的关系。临床医生为特定人群服务时，有责任尽量减少资源的使用量。最小化的资源使用有助于提高可持续性。在可持续性的方面，资源的含义不仅包括金钱。

　　减少浪费和提高可持续性之间的关系如图3.1所示。减少医疗卫生保健中的浪费有立竿见影的收益，它可以释放医疗资源并用于治疗更多的人。然而，还有其他长远获益，不仅是来自于减少医疗浪费，也因为可持续水平的提高。

　　为了妥善管理人群现有的资源，从事群医学的医生不是简单地削减预算，还需要减少浪费并提高可持续性。临床医生必须避免浪费时间，无论是临床医生还是患者的时间，以及不必要的碳资源消耗。

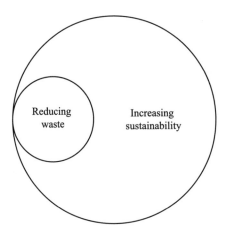

Figure 3.1 The relationship between waste and sustainability

Down with *muda*

In the absence of new resources, those who manage healthcare, most of whom are clinicians, must obtain greater value from the resources available in order to meet increasing need and demand. One way to obtain greater value is to reduce waste. In this situation, there is much to learn from Toyota's success, which is due to an obsession with:

- *kaizan, the relentless pursuit of better quality, and mass customisation, the analogue of personalised medicine;*
- *the eradication of muda, or waste, which Toyota define as "...any activity, service, or supply that consumes time, money, and other resources, but creates no value."* (1)
- *The Toyota formula, which can be applied to health services* (2)*, is: Work done＝Work that produces value＋Waste*

It was Taiichi Ohno, one of the driving forces behind Toyota, who created the obsession with muda or waste. He identified seven categories of waste in industrial systems, which are relevant to healthcare:

1. Overproduction;
2. Time on hand (waiting) ;
3. Stock on hand (inventory) ;

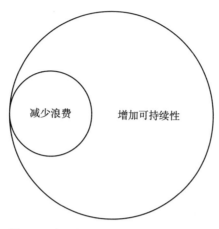

图3.1 减少浪费与可持续性之间的关系

避免浪费

在缺乏新资源的情况下，从事医疗卫生保健的专业人员（其中许多是临床医生）必须从现有资源中获得更大的价值，以满足日益增长的卫生服务需求。获得更大价值的方法之一是减少浪费。在这种情况下，丰田的成功有很多值得学习的地方，其坚持的几点包括：

- 改善（kaizan），对更高质量和大规模定制（类似于个性化医疗）的不懈追求。
- 消除浪费，所谓"浪费"丰田将其定义为"……任何消耗时间、金钱和其他资源但没有创造价值的活动、服务或供应。"[1]
- 丰田公式可以应用于医疗卫生保健服务[2]，即：

已完成的工作＝创造价值的工作＋浪费

大野耐一是丰田幕后推手之一，他创造了消除浪费的理念。他提出了工业系统中的7个浪费类别，与医疗卫生保健具有共性：

1. 生产过剩；
2. 现有的时间（等待）；
3. 现有的库存（滞存）；

4. Waste of movement;

5. Defective products;

6. Transportation;

7. Processing.

Ohno's work, and the concept of 'lean thinking' (3) which flowed from it, are of central importance to those who pay for, or manage, health services. Indeed, Ohno's seven categories of waste have been adapted and expanded in a book by Toussaint, Gerard and Womack (4), specifically aimed at healthcare professionals (see Box 3.1).

Box 3.1　Eight types of waste in healthcare (4)

- Defect: making errors, inspecting work already done for error;
- Waiting: for test results to be delivered, for an appointment, for a bed, for a release of paperwork;
- Motion: searching for supplies, fetching drugs from another room, looking for proper forms;
- Transportation: taking patients through miles of corridors, from one test to the next unnecesarily, transferring patients to new rooms or units, carrying trays of tools between rooms;
- Overproduction: excessive diagnostic testing, unnecessary treatment;
- Overprocessing: a patient being asked the same question three times, unnecessary forms, nurses writing everything in a chart instead of noting exceptions;
- Inventory: (too much or too little); overstocked drugs expiring on the shelf, under-stocked surgical supplies delaying procedures while staff go in search of needed items;
- Talent: failing to listen to employee ideas for innovation.

The magnitude of waste is huge. In an important article, Don Berwick estimated that the cost of waste 'exceeds 20% of total health care expenditure' (5). The six types of waste he identified are:

- *Overtreatment*;
- *Failures of care coordination*;
- *Failures in execution of care processes*;
- *Administrative complexity*;
- *Pricing failures*;
- *Fraud and abuse*.

4．运转过程的损耗；

5．残次品；

6．交通运输；

7．流程设置。

大野耐一的工作，以及由此产生的"精益思维"[3]概念，对于卫生服务的支付者或管理者来说非常重要。事实上，大野耐一的七类浪费已经被托桑、杰拉德和沃玛克[4]采纳并应用于医疗卫生领域（专栏3.1）。

专栏3.1　医疗卫生保健中的八种浪费[4]

- 损失：工作失误，为检查纠正错误所付出的代价。
- 等待：等待测试结果，等待预约、床位、文件公布。
- 行动：寻找物资，从其他房间取药，寻找合适的单据。
- 转运：带患者穿过数英里长的走廊，不必要地进行一个又一个检查，将患者转移到新的房间或单元，在房间之间搬运放工具的托盘。
- 生产过剩：过度诊断测试，不必要的治疗。
- 过度处理：患者同一个问题被问了3次，填写不必要的表格，护士把所有的东西都写在图表上而非仅对异常情况进行记录。
- 现有库存：太多或太少；库存货架上积压了过期的药品，当医务人员寻找所需的物品时，手术用品又库存不足，耽误了手术。
- 人才：未能听取员工的创新想法。

浪费的体量是巨大的。唐·贝里克在一篇重要文章中估计，浪费的成本"超过了医疗卫生总支出的20%"。[5]他确定的六类浪费是：

- 过度治疗；
- 医疗服务中的协作不足；
- 医疗服务过程中执行失误；
- 冗杂的行政管理；
- 定价不合理；
- 欺瞒和滥用。

High-value healthcare involves getting the right patients to the right service and the right treatment done right first time. When taking decisions about what is 'right', lower-value activities need to be identified and excluded. It is also essential to identify and reduce waste, even when the right interventions are being delivered safely and at high quality to the right patients.

Clinicians responsible for serving a population need to minimize waste for two main reasons:

they have a responsibility to the population providing the resources for healthcare not to waste those resources, which could otherwise to release resources so that more people in the population can be treated.

Eight questions to help clinicians identify and minimise waste are shown in Box 3.2.

Box 3.2 Questions to identify waste in health services (4)

Can we make more use of buildings and equipment?

Do we need to carry as much stock?

Can the numbers of non-clinical staff be reduced?

Can the waste of clinician and patient time be reduced?

Is care being delivered in the right place?

Could care be provided by less highly paid staff?

Can we use cheaper drugs and equipment?

Can we prevent waste of human resources?

Question 1: Can we make more use of buildings and equipment?

In most countries, hospitals serve small populations of 100,000-300,000 people. This pattern of development was initiated in an era in when:

- *there was little specialisation other than that between medical and surgical specialties;*
- *car ownership was low;*
- *medical technology, such as imaging technology, was much simpler and less expensive than it is today;*
- *the mobile phone had not even been imagined.*

高价值的群医学就是要让正确的患者获得正确的服务，并在正确的时间进行正确的治疗。当决定什么才算是"正确的"时，需要确定并排除那些低价值的活动。确定和减少浪费也非常重要，即使是在安全高质量地向正确的患者提供正确的干预措施时也应如此。

为人群提供服务的临床医生需要减少浪费，主要有以下两个原因：

● 他们有责任为人群提供卫生资源，且不应浪费，因为这些资源本来也可以用于其他公共服务，如教育或社会服务；

● 释放资源，使更多有需要的人都能够得到治疗。

帮助临床医生识别和减少浪费的8个问题，如专栏3.2所示。

专栏3.2　用于识别医疗卫生服务中的浪费问题[4]

● 我们能否更充分地利用场所空间和设备器材？
● 我们需要多少库存？
● 能否减少非临床医务人员的数量？
● 能否减少对临床医生和患者时间的浪费？
● 是在正确的地方提供了医疗服务吗？
● 医疗服务是否可以由薪酬稍低的员工们来提供？
● 我们能否使用更便宜的药品和设备器材？
● 我们能否防止人力资源浪费？

问题1：我们能否更充分地利用场所空间和设备器材？

在大多数国家，医院为10万至30万人的小规模人群提供服务。这种发展模式始于那个时代：

● 除了内科和外科专业之外，几乎没有其他专科；

● 有车的人很少；

● 医疗技术，如成像技术，比现在简单得多，也便宜得多；

● 移动电话尚未问世。

Today, we have a configuration of health services in which there are too many hospitals with under-utilised buildings and equipment. The considerable growth in the size of hospitals during the last 50 years has largely been characterised by development in isolation and development in competition — the 'medical arms race' — 'St Elsewhere's has just bought a CT scanner; we have to have one too. ' Not every hospital needs to provide every specialty and every piece of equipment. For hospitals to give up a specialty or to choose not to develop a specialty requires strong clinical leadership. Clinicians practising population medicine to be able to justify and explain that it is in the best interests of the population served, to whom they are accountable, for some members of that population to have to travel further for certain services such that resources are not used in the unnecessary duplication of services. Saving the resources entailed in duplication will enable a greater number of patients to be treated; fortunately, this strategy is also often in the best interests of the individual patient.

Question 2: Do we need to carry as much stock?

In 2005, 574 different head and socket combinations were used in [hip replacement] operations in England and Wales. It seems implausible that meaningful data can be gathered, or that money can be saved through bulk purchase, when such a number of products and supplies is used in this way. (6)

Just-in-time delivery of the equipment needed was one of the great achievements of the Toyota production systems, and provides much useful learning for health services. In contrast, most health services buy too much equipment of too many types and store it for too long.

Such waste can be prevented partly by improving procurement practices, but staff responsible for procurement do not act in isolation. They tend to buy what clinicians want, seeking the lowest possible price but not necessarily questioning the added value of the new item that a clinician has requested. Indeed, the rigorous appraisal of requests relating to clinical procurement must be done by the clinician leading on population medicine, who needs to persuade colleagues that it is not only the cost of new medical devices that wastes resources but also the costs of storage, stock control and the disposal of unused or unwanted devices. Pharmacies represent a model of good stock control that other hospital departments can follow.

目前，在我们的医疗卫生资源的配置中，有太多医院的场所空间和设备器材利用不足。在过去50年中，医院规模的显著增长主要表现为在孤立中发展和在竞争中发展，即"医疗军备竞赛"——"其他医院买了一台CT机，我们也不得不买一台"。不是每一家医院都需要提供每一种专科和每一种设备。对于医院来说，放弃某项专科或选择不发展某个专科，都需要具备强大的临床领导才能。从事群医学的临床医生应该有能力向所服务的人群说明：为了保证群体利益最大化，一些人需要前往其他医疗机构获得特定的医疗服务，以避免因为不必要的重复服务而过度使用资源。节省重复性工作中的资源将使更多需要治疗的患者能够得到救治。幸运的是，这种策略通常也符合患者个人的最大利益。

问题2：我们需要多少库存？

2005年，英格兰和威尔士的（髋关节置换）手术中使用了574种不同的头窝组合。当使用了如此多的产品和用品时，想要收集有意义的数据或通过批量采购节省开支是不切实际的。[6]

能够及时交付所需设备器材是丰田生产系统的一大成绩，为医疗卫生领域提供了许多有益借鉴。相比之下，在医疗卫生领域，普遍存在购买过多种类的设备器材，以及闲置时间过长的问题。

通过改进采购方法可以在一定程度上防止这种浪费，但负责采购的工作人员不应独自行动。他们虽倾向于购买临床医生想要的东西，并寻求可能的最低价格，但不一定会质疑临床医生所要求新产品的附加值。相反，应该由群医学领域的临床医生来严格评估与临床采购相关的申请。该临床医生必须说服同事们认识到：资源的浪费不仅存在于购买新医疗器械的花费，还存在于存储、控制库存以及处理未使用或不需要设备的成本等方面。在此，药房展现了一种良好的库存控制模式，医院的其他部门可以效仿。

Question 3: Can the numbers of non-clinical staff be reduced?

Contrary to popular belief, administrative staff do not create their own work.

- *The work of staff in the central management of a health service is created by outside agencies, which impose certain tasks or require specific information on a regular basis.*
- *Much of the work of administrative staff in clinical areas is created by clinicians; some of the administrative tasks may be unnecessary tasks but only because clinicians have not addressed the need to make the work of 'clinical microsystems' leaner.*

A clinical microsystem is a small group of people who work together on a regular basis to provide care to discrete subpopulations of patients. It has clinical and business aims, linked processes, and a shared information environment, and it produces performance outcomes. Microsystems evolve over time and are often embedded in larger organizations. They are complex adaptive systems, and as such they must do the primary work associated with core aims, meet the needs of their members, and maintain themselves over time as clinical units. (7)

Even teams that work well together may undertake lower-value activities that have crept into their clinical practice over the years, and which need to be eradicated, such as:

- *collecting data which no-one uses;*
- *handovers done on paper that could be done digitally;*
- *failing to involve the patient as a key member of the team.*

Question 4: Can the waste of clinician and patient time be reduced?

For clinicians, time is the scarcest resource: it is finite and once expended cannot be recovered. Unfortunately, much of a clinician's time is wasted. Often, the job of a clinician involves more than encounters with patients during clinical practice. It can encompass management, education and research, and all aspects of a clinician's job, including clinical practice can incur a waste of time.

问题3：能否减少非临床医务人员数量？

与大众认识不同的是，行政管理人员不能自己创建工作内容。

- 只有当某些外部机构需要定期开展某些工作或需要某些具体信息时，才有了医疗卫生保健核心管理工作人员的工作任务。
- 临床管理人员的大部分工作是由临床医生提出的；某些管理任务可能是不必要的，只是由于临床医生尚未能精简"临床微系统"的工作。

所谓的临床微系统是指：一小群人定期地共同为离群、散居的患者提供医疗卫生保健。该系统有临床和业务目标、相互关联的流程和共享的信息环境，并产生绩效结果。微系统随着时间的推移而发展，并嵌入更大的组织中。它们是复杂的适应性系统，因此它们必须完成与核心目标相关的主要工作，满足其成员的需求，并随着时间的推移保持自己作为临床单元的地位。[7]

即使是合作良好的团队，也可能会从事一些低价值的活动。这些低价值活动已在过去的几年里渗透到了临床实践中，有待根除，例如：

- 收集无人使用的数据；
- 仍采用纸质交接可数字化的工作；
- 未能让患者成为团队的关键成员。

问题4：能否减少临床医生和患者在时间上的浪费？

对临床医生来说，时间是最稀缺的资源：时间是有限的，且一旦被使用就无法再生。不幸的是，临床医生的许多时间都被浪费了。通常，临床医生的工作不仅是在临床工作中诊治患者，还包括管理、教育和科学研究工作。临床医生的这些工作，包括临床实践，虽然本质上是有价值的，但都可能导致时间的浪费。

Waste of time in management

Many physicians are reimbursed for half a day to recognise the time spent in managing resources, but much of this can be considered a "waste", undertaking activities such as:

- *writing a plan that has no possibility of realisation*;
- *contributing to projects that are poorly managed or do not deliver the anticipated outputs*;
- *meetings without purpose or conclusion.*

All clinicians are more than likely to have their own ideas about what constitutes a waste of time, but their perceptions may not be shared. Attendance at a management meeting may be considered a waste of time by a clinician, but regarded as high value by a manager. Independent evaluation is required to determine which of the two perceptions is correct: the clinician because the meeting was unfocused and unproductive, or the manager because the clinician came to a meeting that was of value but with the wrong attitude.

Waste of time in education

Education can have benefits, but it is always associated with a cost. Education is of low value or represents a waste of time if:

- *the intervention has been selected in accordance with the clinician's desire rather than through a formal assessment of learning needs — there is evidence that if clinicians are interested in a topic, they will seek the learning they need*(8); *expenditure on formal training should be reserved only for areas of clinical practice in which the clinician needs to improve the quality of care being delivered or as part of a planned innovation*;
- *the educational methods employed are not supported by evidence of effectiveness; lectures are usually of low value.*

Waste of time in research

The value of investing public money in research is hotly debated, but most countries in Europe and North America now realise that it is important to develop an economy based on knowledge rather than one based on exporting agricultural products or manufactured goods.

在管理中浪费的时间

考虑到在管理资源上花费的时间，许多临床医生可以得到半天的补偿。但如从事以下活动时，这"半天的补偿"也可以被视为是"浪费"。这些活动包括：

- 编写不可能实现的计划；
- 参与管理不善或无法交付预期成果的项目；
- 参加无目的或无结论的会议。

临床医生对什么是浪费时间很可能有自己的认识，但看法不一定一致。临床医生可能会认为参加管理会议是在浪费时间，但管理者却认为会议很有价值。临床医生认为会议没有重点也没有产出；管理者认为临床医生参加的会议有其价值所在，但参会医生态度敷衍了事（因此无法从中有所获益），这两种观点哪一种正确，需要分别从不同角度独立评估分析。

在教育中浪费的时间

教育可以带来效益，但亦有其成本。教育在下列情况可视为价值很低或是浪费时间：

- 学习内容的选择是根据临床医生的主观意愿而非通过对学习需求的正式评估——有证据表明，如果临床医生对某个主题感兴趣，他们就会根据自己的需求学习[8]；正式培训的支出应仅用于临床医生对医疗质量的提升或作为创新规划的一部分；
- 没有证据可证明所使用的教育方法是有效的；讲座的价值通常很低。

在研究中浪费的时间

将公共资金投资于研究一直饱受争议，但欧洲和北美的大多数国家现在都意识到，经济发展靠的是知识，而非出口农产品或工业成品。

Once the funding agency has allocated the financial resources to the clinical researcher, there is much that could be done to increase the level of productivity in research (9). Chalmers and Glasziou identified waste at all four stages of the research process (see Box 3.3).

Box 3.3 Avoidable waste in the clinical research process (9)

- Choosing the wrong question for research
- Doing studies that are unnecessary or poorly designed
- Failing to publish results promptly or not at all
- Producing biased or unusable reports of research

Chalmers and Glasziou concluded that:

...action to address this waste is needed now because it has human as well as economic consequences. (9)

Waste of time in clinical practice

Clinical practice is of high value, but within the course of clinical work the time of clinicians is wasted if:

- *the patient's notes are missing;*
- *key data, such as laboratory results, are not available;*
- *there is unnecessary waiting time, such as between operations in theatre.*

Wasting the time of patients

The problems that incur a waste of time for clinicians can also waste the time of patients, especially as there is increasing recognition that patients have to make a significant contribution to their own care even if they do not have to pay for the cost of it. The concept of a 'treatment burden' draws attention to the four types of 'work' that patients with complex problems have to undertake (see Box 3.4). Considering the burden of work for patients receiving care, it is important that clinicians and other healthcare professionals give careful consideration to the ways in which patients' time is wasted and how this may be ameliorated.

一旦资助机构将财政资源分配给临床研究人员，在提高生产力水平和减少研究中的浪费方面有很多工作可以做[9]。查默斯和格拉斯乔发现在研究过程的4个阶段都可能产生浪费（专栏3.3）。

专栏3.3 临床研究过程中可避免的浪费[9]

- 选择错误的研究问题。
- 进行不必要或设计不当的研究项目。
- 未能及时或根本不发表其研究结果。
- 得出有偏倚的或无用的研究报告。

查默斯和格拉斯乔的结论认为：

……现在需要采取行动解决浪费问题，因为它会给人和经济带来影响。[9]

在临床实践中浪费时间

临床实践具有很高价值。但在临床工作过程中，如果有以下情况则是在浪费时间：

- 缺失了患者的有关记录；
- 无法获取关键数据，如实验室结果；
- 不必要的等待时间，如手术室中两次手术之间的等待时间。

浪费患者的时间

导致临床医生浪费时间的问题同样会浪费患者的时间，特别是随着越来越多的人认识到，即使患者不必支付任何费用，他们也需要为自己的健康有所作为。"治疗的负担"这一概念使人们注意到具有复合型问题的患者自身必须承担的4种"工作"（专栏3.4）。考虑到照护患者的工作负担，临床医生和其他医疗卫生专业人员应仔细考虑患者的时间是以什么方式被浪费的以及如何改进。

Box 3.4 Work undertaken by patients with complex problems during treatment (10)

- Learning About Treatments and Their Consequences: Sensemaking Work
- Engaging with Others/Mobilizing Resources: Participation Work
- Adhering to Treatments and Lifestyle Changes: Enacting Work
- Monitoring the Treatments: Appraisal Work

Question 5: Is care being delivered in the right place?

Many patients receive care at healthcare facilities where the levels of staffing and other resources are of an intensity unnecessary for good patient outcomes. Examples of patients usually cared for in secondary care facility who could be cared for elsewhere are given below.

- *Patients, usually older people, who have recovered from the acute phase of their disease but cannot be discharged because they are too disabled to return home and yet cannot be found a place in a nursing home. This situation is of concern not only for those who manage or pay for care but also for the patients who are at high risk of hospital-acquired infection, institutionalisation, and malnutrition;*
- *Patients who attend a clinic with a problem that could have been resolved if their primary care clinician had had a convenient and fast method of accessing the expertise of the specialist, such as via an email, a 'phone call or a video link;*
- *People who die in hospital who could have been supported to die at home.*

Question 6: Could care be provided by less highly paid staff?

Highly trained staff are scarce and expensive to train. It is a waste of skill if highly trained staff undertake tasks that could be managed equally well by other staff who have not had the same level of training but whose training has enabled them to carry out a specific range of tasks. Less highly trained staff are able to undertake repetitive tasks with greater attention to detail and to obtain better results than those achieved by the most highly trained staff for whom such tasks are not relevant to their core function.

专栏3.4 具有复合型问题的患者在治疗期间需要做的事情[10]

- 了解治疗及其后果：感知。
- 与他人交流/筹集资源：参与。
- 坚持治疗和改变生活方式：配合。
- 监测治疗：评估。

问题5：是否在正确的地点提供了卫生服务？

许多患者在医疗机构接受医疗卫生保健，但该机构中人员和资源的配备对于实现患者的良好预后并非必要。下面给出了通常在二级医疗机构就医的患者，而这些患者本可以在其他地方就诊的例子。

- 已经从疾病急性期恢复、但由于行动不便无法居家疗养却又找不到康复疗养机构而不能出院的患者，通常是老年人。这种情况不仅关系到那些管理或支付费用的人，也关系到那些可有较高风险发生院内感染、长期住在养老机构和发生营养不良的患者；
- 到诊所就诊的患者的问题可以通过下述方式得到解决：患者的初级卫生保健医生能通过电子邮件、电话或视频等方便快捷的方式、从专科医学处获得相关的专业知识；
- 本可以在家中接受临终关怀的患者却在医院里去世。

问题6：是否可以让薪酬较低的员工来提供医疗服务？

训练有素的医务人员人数稀少且培训成本高，如果他们所承担的工作本可在确保质量的同时由未经高级培训人员开展，会造成一种技术上的浪费。这些接受培训较少的医务人员即便没有接受足够完备的培训，仍能完成一些特定任务。培训程度较低的工作人员能够执行重复性任务，更加注重细节，并取得比培训程度最高的工作人员更好的结果，也因为这些任务往往并不是接受过高级培训的医务人员的核心职务。

Question 7: Can we use cheaper equipment and drugs?

The key question when considering waste in relation to equipment and drugs is why pay more than is necessary?Costs can be reduced by:

- *skilful procurement*;
- *bulk purchase*;
- *the use of generic rather than branded drugs*;
- *'making' rather than 'buying'* ;
- *sharing services*.

These activities are ethically important because they reduce waste, increase productivity and release resources for clinical care. In a significant policy commitment in the *White Paper, Equity and Excellence: Liberating the NHS* (11), the Government stated that 'we will pay drug companies according to the value of new medicines', a policy referred to as value-based pricing.(12)

Moreover, there are often alternatives to interventions, and the clinician can choose the one that is more cost-effective. The aim of cost-effectiveness analysis is to identify the lowest cost option.

...[cost-effectiveness analysis] compares the costs of alternative ways of achieving a given objective. Where two or more interventions are found to achieve the same level of benefits, the intervention with the least cost is the most cost-effective alternative.(13)

Cost-effectiveness analysis(CEA) is used to address questions of technical efficiency. It is applied in situations where a choice between at least two options with the same goal must be made. That is, given that a particular goal is to be achieved for a fixed budget, CEA can provide a response to the question, 'What is the best way to obtain that goal?' (14)

Once cost-benefit or cost-utility analysis has been used to assess whether an intervention offers good value, cost-effectiveness analysis allows the comparison of two or more methods of achieving the result.

问题7：我们能否使用更便宜的设备器材和药品？

在考虑与设备和药品有关的浪费时，关键问题是为什么要支付更多不必要的费用？以下方式可以降低成本：

- 有技巧地采购；
- 批量采购；
- 使用仿制药而非原研药；
- "制造"而非"购买"；
- 共享医疗卫生保健。

这些行动减少了浪费，提高了生产力，并为临床医疗提供了资源，从伦理角度看非常重要。在《公平与卓越：解放NHS》[11] 白皮书中的一项重要政策承诺中，政府表示，"我们将根据新药的价值向制药公司付款"，这一政策被称为基于价值的定价。[12]

另外，在存在可替代的方法的情况下，临床医生可以选择更具成本效益的方法。成本-效果分析的目的是确定最低成本的选择。

……［成本-效果分析］比较了实现既定目标的各种备选方案的成本。如果发现两种或两种以上的干预措施能够获得相同的效益水平，则成本最低的干预措施是最具成本-效果的替代方案。[13]

成本-效果分析（CEA）用于解决技术效率问题。它适用于必须在至少两个具有相同目标的选项之间进行选择的情况。也就是说，考虑到固定预算要实现特定目标，CEA可以回答这样一个问题："实现该目标的最佳方式是什么？"[14]

使用成本-效益分析或成本-效用分析评估干预措施是否具有良好价值后，可以使用成本-效果分析就可以对两种或更多种干预措施进行比较，看哪一种方法更可达到预期的结果。

If cost-benefit analysis demonstrates the value of revascularization of the coronary arteries, cost-effectiveness analysis enables two methods, coronary artery bypass grafting and stenting, to be compared.

If cost-benefit analysis demonstrates that the treatment of less severe depression appears to have benefit, cost-effectiveness analysis can be used to answer the question of whether it is less costly to use drugs or cognitive therapy.

Irrespective of the answer to questions posed during cost-effectiveness analysis, there is a supplementary question concerning costliness, for example:

- *Which drug is the least costly?*
- *Is face-to-face or online consultation less costly?*

Such questions are often more subtle and less clear-cut than would appear at first sight. There may be small differences in the magnitude of the benefits and harms of each option, or in the probabilities of good and bad outcomes. The decisions about which of the options to choose involve not only a cost comparison but also a judgement about which of the trade-offs associated with each option is preferred in the current context. The simplest type of comparison is that regarding the use of a generic drug when compared with the proprietary product because both interventions are identical in effect but different in price. However, there is evidence that many clinicians do not choose the cheapest option in this situation.

Question 8: Can we prevent waste of human resources?

Demanding though it may be to work on the Toyota production line, that task is much simpler than those associated with clinical practice. For many people, the admonition not to waste the untapped potential of professionals would be interpreted as a call to provide more and better quality continuing professional development. However, greater challenges face the clinician responsible for delivering a service to a population:

- *staff retention and turnover — investment in training does not realise much value if a high proportion of those trained, such as nurses, leave within five years;*
- *burnout — the largest waste of professional talent, particularly when considering the case of clinicians.*

如果成本－效益分析可以证明冠状动脉血运重建的价值，那么成本－效果分析就可以比较冠状动脉搭桥术和支架置入术这两种方法。

如果成本－效益分析表明，治疗轻度抑郁症可获得效益，那么成本－效果分析可以用来回答下述问题：在药物或认知疗法二者间，哪种方法成本更低。

无论成本－效果分析过程中所提问题的答案是什么，都有一个关于成本的补充问题，例如：

- 哪种药最便宜？
- 面对面咨询和在线咨询，哪一种的成本更低？

这类问题往往比乍看上去更微妙也更模糊。每种选择的利弊或结果好坏上可能仅有微小差别。决定选择哪种方案不仅涉及其成本比较，还需权衡每个选项的交互关系，才能做出当下最适宜的选择。最简单的比较方式是把常用药与专利药相比，因为两种药物的疗效相同而价格相异。而在这种情况下，临床医生并不一定总会选择那些最便宜的。

问题8：我们能否防止人力资源的浪费？

虽然在丰田生产线上可能对工作要求很高，但比起临床实践相关的任务来说要简单得多。对很多人来说，告诫不要浪费专业人员尚未开发的潜力，将被解读为呼吁提供更多、更高质量的持续专业发展。但是，这对践行群医学的临床医生来说是一个很大的挑战：

- 医务人员的留用率和离职率——如果大部分受培训人员（如护士）在五年内离职，用于培训的投资就没有得到回报；
- 职业倦怠——这是对专业人才的最大浪费，尤其是临床医生。

Burnout is usually identified by three major symptoms: emotional exhaustion, depersonalisation, and decreased sense of self-efficacy. But burnout, we believe is also a euphemism for what many physicians experience as a crisis of meaning and identity. Burnout is the index of dislocation between what people are and what they have to do. It represents an erosion in values, dignity, spirit, and will-and erosion of the human soul.(15)

The main concern about burnout is not necessarily the loss of workforce and the waste of resources involved in workforce training, but that healthcare professionals can begin to work in a way that is detrimental to the service, annoying for colleagues and upsetting for any patients they may encounter. As pressure increases to meet rising need and demand in a context of no new resources while also continuing to improve quality and safety, in the absence of good leadership, the prevalence of burnout will increase. Indeed, the prevalence of burnout may be worsened by the need for managers to impose what has been called the target culture. The impact of burnout in the United States of America could be serious, especially in the context of implementing universal coverage, but it is by no means a problem unique to the USA.

For reform to achieve its goal of providing all residents access to high quality medical care, efforts to identify and address the controllable factors contributing to burnout among physicians are needed.(16)

Even when burnout is not a problem experienced by physicians and other healthcare professionals, staff can behave in other ways that are counter-productive and difficult to deal with such as the subtle withdrawal of enthusiasm. In developing a health service for a population, it is essential not only to be concerned about strategy and systems, but also to consider and empathise with the situation of frontline staff. The words of Viscount Slim, perhaps Britain's most respected leader in the Second World War, are resonant here. He recognised the need to support personnel in a way that enables them to apply their character traits to the fulfilment of their responsibilities:

...the high quality of the individual soldier, his morale, toughness and discipline, his acceptance of hardship and his ability to move on his own feet and to look after himself.(17)

职业倦怠通常有3个主要症状：情绪耗竭、人格解体和自我效能感下降。但是，我们相信它也是许多医生都经历的"人生意义和自我认同危机"的委婉说法。职业倦怠显示了"我是谁，我该做什么"二者之间的混乱。它代表着对人类价值观、尊严、精神和意志等方面受到的侵蚀——以及对灵魂的侵蚀。[15]

职业倦怠的主要问题不一定是劳动力流失和职业培训的资源浪费，而是医护人员开始以一种不良方式工作，不仅使同事感到恼火，也让被服务对象感到失望。在没有新资源的情况下，持续改进质量和安全性以满足不断增长的卫生服务需要和需求，会导致压力不断增加；同时在没有良好领导的情况下，职业倦怠将更加普遍。确切来说，由于管理者强制实行所谓的"目标文化"，普遍性的职业倦怠可能会进一步恶化。美国职业倦怠的影响可能很严重，尤其是在实施全民健康覆盖的情况下，但此问题绝非美国独有。

为了实现向所有居民提供高质量医疗服务的改革目标，需要努力确定和解决导致医生职业倦怠的可控因素。[16]

即使临床医生和其他医疗卫生专业人员没有遇到职业倦怠问题，员工也会以其他形式表现出逆反或难以应对的行为，如难以觉察到的工作热情降低等。在为某人群订制医疗卫生项目时，虽然策略和体系非常重要，但是也应该考虑和理解那些一线工作人员的状况。作为可能是英国在第二次世界大战中最受尊敬的领导人，Viscount Slim子爵的话在这里引起了共鸣。他认为，需要设计一种激励机制，使每个人的品性与其所履行的职责有效契合：

……每位高素质的士兵，他的士气、坚韧和纪律感，他应对困难、自立和照顾自己的能力。[17]

■ Reducing waste contributes to increased sustainability

Sustainability is a key concept for the 21st century, and the reduction of waste increases the sustainability of any organisation. However, sustainability covers a much broader range of topics than the reduction of waste, and it is of central importance to population medicine, although healthcare in general needs to become much more sustainable (18).

Although the waste reduction is important, it is not sufficient when identifying ways in which to increase sustainability (and value). The clinician fulfilling responsibilities for population medicine needs to consider the impact of clinical practice on the environment and not just the amount of resources consumed. In the UK, the renal service has set the standard for establishing sustainability as a central concern in clinical practice (19). The change in culture necessary to make sustainability a central concern, and not one at the margins, is one of the most important responsibilities in population medicine. Clinicians who manage healthcare need:

- *to reduce the carbon footprint of their services*;
- *to increase the sustainability of their services.*

Just as more of the same is not the way to meet the challenges of the future, neither is less of the same.

The meaning of 'sustainable development'

Sustainable development has been described as 'protecting resources from one generation to the next' (20). However, the term 'sustainable development' is widely used and has different meanings for different people. Originally, the term was taken to have an environmental meaning, such as that shown in Box 3.5.

Box 3.5 The environmental meaning of sustainable development (21)

- Consuming fewer material goods
- Using locally produced goods and services to reduce their carbon emissions from their transportation — this will also contribute to the economic sustainability of local communities
- Ensuring that goods and services are produced in as energy-efficient a way as possible with minimal waste (which is recycled)
- Ensuring material goods (such as washing machines, TVs, fridges, etc.) are themselves energy efficient

■ 减少浪费有助于提高可持续性

可持续发展是21世纪的重要概念，任何组织减少浪费均可提高可持续性。然而除了减少浪费，可持续性涵盖主题范围更广阔，并且这对群医学至关重要，尽管医疗卫生领域需要提高可持续性。[18]

虽然减少浪费很重要，但在识别提高可持续性（和价值）的手段时，这是不够的。承担群医学职责的临床医生需要考虑临床实践对环境的影响，而不仅是资源的消耗量。在英国，肾脏服务中心已经制定了标准，将可持续性作为临床实践的核心问题[19]。进行必要的文化建设，使可持续发展成为核心而非边缘内容，这是群医学最重要的职责之一。从事医疗管理工作的临床医生需要做到以下几点：

- 减少其服务的碳足迹；
- 提高其服务的整体可持续性。

无论如何，都不能沿用以前的方法来应对未来的挑战。

"可持续发展"的含义

"可持续发展"指的是"一代又一代地保护后代资源"[20]。尽管"可持续发展"一词被广泛使用，但不同的人有不同的理解。最初，这个词被认为有环境方面的含义，如专栏3.5所示。

专栏3.5　可持续发展的环境含义[21]

- 减少物资消耗。
- 利用当地生产的商品和提供的服务，减少交通运输带来的碳排放——这也有助于当地经济的可持续发展。
- 确保生产产品和提供服务时，尽可能节约能源、减少浪费（回收利用）。
- 确保物资（如洗衣机、电视机、冰箱等）本身是节能的。

The term, however, now has a broader meaning, perhaps best expressed in the following quotation from *The Lancet's* Global Health Commission:

> *The concept of sustainable development was formulated to address issues of intergenerational equity in resource availability. It has been condemned as lacking definition and conceptual rigour.*
>
> *However, it offers the possibility of fundamental changes to the way we consume and produce, the way we arrange our functionally fragmented institutions, and the way we distribute resources globally and locally. Most importantly, sustainable development not only posits environmental degradation and poverty as interconnected issues, but it gives an example of how mainstream politics might be brought into a debate that demands a complete rethink of our institutions, resources, and environmental outcome, and also assumes that thee issues can be solved with political will.(22)*

Although sustainability now encompasses many issues, carbon and its effect on climate change are of vital concern to healthcare professionals given that climate change is one of the principal threats to global health in the 21st century. This may be the reason why this issue tends to have the greatest potential for motivating frontline staff. Thus, implementing a concern for sustainability can be encapsulated within a carbon reduction strategy. The NHS Carbon Reduction Strategy for England was first published in 2009. Eight key areas for action were identified, including energy and carbon management.

> *...NHS scenarios in a low carbon world need to be developed to understand the different ways healthcare delivery must be shaped for a low carbon future. The impact this will have on models of care, and how to develop and promote low carbon pathways, must be understood.*
>
> *This strategy sets the ambition for the NHS to play a leading and innovative role in ensuring the shift to a low carbon society.(18)*

The NHS Sustainable Development Unit(SDU) produces a range of materials for staff, highlighting the short-and long-term benefits of carbon reduction. It emphasises that the NHS must meet the targets enshrined in the Climate Change Act 2008(see Box 3.6), but by so doing many health and financial co-benefits will also be realised.

然而，这个词现在有了更广泛的含义，以下《柳叶刀》全球健康委员会的引文或许最能表达这一点：

提出可持续发展的概念是为了解决资源可得性的代际公平问题。它被责难缺乏定义和概念上的严谨性。

然而，它为我们在消费和生产的方式、在安排职能分散的机构以及在全球和地方如何分配资源的方式等方面都提供了根本性改变的可能。最重要的是，可持续发展不仅将环境退化和贫困视为相互关联的问题，而且还提供了一个实例，说明如何将主流政治也纳入对我们的体制、资源和环境结果进行全面反思的辩论并假设这些问题是可以通过政治意愿来解决的。[22]

尽管目前可持续性包含许多问题，但"碳及其对气候变化的影响"是医疗卫生专业人员极为关注的问题，因为气候变化是21世纪全球健康的主要威胁之一。这也许就是为什么这个问题最有可能调动那些在一线工作的员工积极性的原因。因此，对可持续性的关注可以包含在碳减排的战略中。NHS碳减排战略于2009年首次发布。确定了8个重点行动领域，包括能源和碳管理。

……在低碳世界中，需要发展不同的NHS场景，以了解该怎样通过不同的医疗卫生途径以实现低碳化未来。必须了解这对不同照护模式的影响，以及如何开发和促进低碳化的医疗路径。

这一战略确立了NHS在确保向低碳社会转型方面发挥引领和创新作用的雄心。[18]

NHS的可持续发展部门（SDU）为其员工制作了一系列材料，突出了碳减排的短期和长期效益。它强调NHS必须达到《2008年气候变化法案》（专栏3.6）中规定的目标，此举也将同时实现许多健康和财政方面的效益。

■ Reducing the carbon footprint of healthcare

In Chapter 2, the drive to increase value was described in terms of being able to release resources — whether those resources are time, staff or money — for reallocation to meet some other need. However, this presupposes that the only relevant currency is money, whereas another important currency is carbon.

The NHS, as for all other organisations both public and private, needs to reduce its carbon footprint. The NHS is the largest public sector contributor to climate change through its carbon emissions (18) —21 million tonnes of CO_2 equivalents ($MtCO_2e$) in 2007. (23)

The main sources contributing to NHS England's carbon footprint are shown in Figure 3.2.

Although the energy used in heating and lighting the buildings of a health service is considerable and responsible for one-fifth of the carbon footprint, it is not the largest contributor. Three-fifths of the NHS' carbon footprint can be attributed to the manufacture, distribution, use and disposal of drugs and equipment, the "tools" of clinical research and practice. Thus, even if every hospital and health centre converted to renewable energy, the NHS would not achieve its challenging targets for carbon reduction (see Box 3.6).

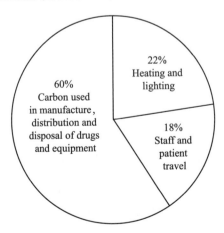

Figure 3.2 Sources contributing to the carbon footprint of NHS England (18)

专栏3.6　英国NHS减少碳排放的目标（基于1990年）[23]

- 至2020年减少34%。
- 至2030年减少64%。
- 至2050年减少80%。

■ 减少医疗卫生的碳足迹

第二章描述了增加价值的驱动力，即为满足更多需求，该如何释放资源——无论是时间、人员还是金钱——并进行重新分配。然而，此前提假设是："钱"是其唯一相关的硬通货，而另一个重要硬通货则是"碳"。

NHS与其他所有公共和私营医疗卫生机构一样，都需要减少其碳足迹。NHS是通过碳排放而对气候变化影响最大的公共部门[18]，其碳排放在2007年达到2100万吨二氧化碳当量（$MtCO_2e$）。[23]

英国NHS碳足迹的主要来源如图3.2所示。

尽管用于医疗卫生机构的供暖和照明能源相当可观，占碳排放量的五分之一，但其并不是碳足迹的最大来源。NHS五分之三的碳足迹可归因于药物、设备以及临床研究和实践"工具"的制造、分销、使用和处置。因此，即使每个医院和医疗中心都转为使用可再生能源，NHS亦无法实现其具有挑战性的碳减排目标（专栏3.6）。

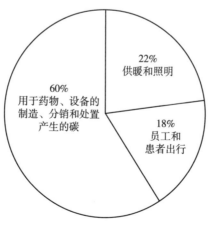

图3.2　英国NHS碳排放量的来源[18]

Despite the fact that it is important to reduce the energy use of healthcare buildings:

- *it is vital to reduce the amount of carbon used during clinical research and practice*;
- *it is necessary to reduce the carbon used during staff and patient travel-this contributes almost as much to the carbon footprint as heating and lighting.*

This is why the emphasis in the *White Paper Equity and Excellence: Liberating the NHS*(11)on reducing the NHS' carbon footprint is not limited to health services using less energy, it also requires clinicians to change the way in which they deliver care.

Carbon will become an increasingly important constraint in the planning and delivery of health services. Already in the UK, hospitals have been given carbon budgets. These budgets will not grow, even if more money should become available; instead carbon budgets will decrease year on year in order to meet the targets set in the NHS England Carbon Reduction Strategy(see Box 3.6).

Unusually for preventive interventions, the payback time for some carbon reduction measures is rapid. In the White Paper, it is anticipated that cash can be released within the same year by 'improving energy efficiency and developing more sustainable forms of delivery'(11).

Sustainable clinical practice

To reduce the NHS' carbon footprint substantially requires a change in the style of clinical practice. Frances Mortimer, Medical Director of the Centre for Sustainable Healthcare, has developed a model of sustainable clinical practice(see Box 3.7).

Box 3.7 Model of sustainable clinical practice(24)

- All clinicians should be involved in prevention, the most sustainable type of health service
- Patient-centred care, for example, sending most laboratory results directly to patients to reduce the number of trips to health centres to collect results
- Leaner pathways, reducing the number of outpatient and follow-up appointments of low or no value
- The consideration of carbon costs as well as financial costs when considering the cose-effectiveness of treatment

Engaging staff in sustainability

Attitudes towards sustainability, and how to address it in a health service, vary. For some healthcare professionals, carbon reduction is an important issue because of

尽管减少医疗卫生机构的能源使用非常重要：

- 在临床研究和实践中，减少碳使用量也至关重要；

- 有必要减少工作人员和患者出行期间使用的碳——其碳足迹几乎与供暖和照明的碳足迹相当。

这就是为什么白皮书《公平与卓越：解放NHS》[11] 中强调减少NHS碳排放量不仅限于提供耗能较少的医疗卫生照护，还要求临床医生改变行医方式。

碳将日益成为医疗卫生规划和供给的制约因素。在英国，医院有其碳预算。即使有更多资金可用，这些预算也不会增长；相反，碳预算将逐年减少，以实现英国NHS碳减排战略中设定的目标（专栏3.6）。

不同寻常的是，对于预防性干预来说，一些碳减排措施的回报很快。白皮书预期，通过"提高能源效率和制定更多可持续的供给模式"，同年即可得到现金收益[11]。

可持续的临床实践

要显著地减少NHS的碳足迹，实质上需要改变临床实践的方式。英国可持续医疗中心主任弗朗西斯·莫蒂默开创了一种可持续的临床实践模式（专栏3.7）。

专栏3.7　可持续临床实践模式

- 所有临床医生都应致力于预防，这是最具有可持续性的卫生服务类型。
- 以患者为中心的照护，例如，将大多数实验室结果直接发送给患者，以减少前往医疗中心拿取结果的次数。
- 精简路径，减少低价值或无价值的门诊和随访预约数量。
- 在考虑治疗的成本－效果时也要考虑碳成本和经济成本。

让员工参与可持续发展

对可持续性的态度以及如何在卫生服务中解决可持续性问题，众说纷纭。对于某些医疗卫生专业人士来说，碳减排是一个重要问题，因为这关乎

concern about their children's future, but others do not believe that climate change is happening. Some staff believe that the health service, or their own part of the health service, is too small to make a difference. However, the experience of the NHS Sustainable Development Unit (SDU) and the Centre for Sustainable Healthcare is that many staff are motivated to change because of the threat of climate change, even those staff who are resistant to appeals to work differently to save money due to the financial plight of the organisation. Suggestions about the ways in which to motivate staff to increase the sustainability of a health service are shown in Box 3.8.

Box 3.8 Ways to motivate staff to increase the sustainability of a health service

- Provide information about the effects of climate change on health
- Describe the factors that contribute to the carbon footprint of a health service
- Ask staff to report what their children are saying about climate change
- Ask how staff are changing their lifestyle to cope with either the threat of climate change or simply the rising cost of energy
- Introduce the concept of 'lean' production, namely, production without waste, because some staff will be motivated by this whatever their views on climate change
- Take part in projects to improve the natural environment of healthcare facilities, for example, the Centre for Sustainable Healthcareruns the NHS Forest, with the aim of planting a tree for every NHS employee

Another way of motivating staff is to provide financial and other incentives. Although It may be difficult to identify all the changes resulting from the implementation of a carbon reduction plan because, for example, the electricity used by the ward cannot be identified separately within a hospital's bill, it is usually possible to identify some measures to monitor the decreased use of resources.

If carbon savings by a ward or health centre can result in some financial reward, so much the better, but it is also important to appeal to the altruism of staff, encouraging them to take action for the good of society, and the next and future generations including their own children.

Adopting a broad approach to sustainability

It is important to adopt a broad approach to sustainability, considering such aspects as:

- *Energy and carbon management*;
- *Procurement and food*;
- *Travel, transport and access*;

孩子的未来；但其他人可能并不相信正在发生的气候变化。一些员工认为，医疗卫生或其自身所从事的医疗项目，由于影响范围太小而很难发挥作用。然而，根据NHS可持续发展部（SDU）和可持续医疗中心的经验，许多员工因气候变化的威胁而有动力做出改变，即使是那些由于所在机构的财务困境而拒绝以不同方式工作以节省资金的员工。关于如何激励员工提高医疗卫生可持续性的方法，见专栏3.8。

专栏3.8　激励员工提高医疗卫生可持续性的方法

- 提供气候变化对健康影响的相关信息。
- 描述影响医疗服务碳排放量的各种因素。
- 请员工就自己孩子对气候变化的看法进行汇报。
- 询问员工如何改变生活方式以应对气候变化的威胁或仅是能源成本的上升（家庭开支的增加）等问题。
- 引入精益生产的概念，即无浪费生产。这是因为无论员工对气候变化的看法如何，某些员工都会为此受到激励。
- 参与改善医疗卫生设施自然环境的项目，例如，可持续医疗中心经营NHS森林，目的是为每一个NHS员工种植一棵树。

激励员工的另一种方式是提供经济和其他方面的激励措施。尽管很难判断由于实施碳减排计划而产生的效果，例如，在医院的账单中无法单独确定病房所消耗的电能，但通常可以采取一些措施来监测资源的利用减少了多少。

如果一个病房或健康中心的碳排放下降能带来一些经济回报，那就更好了。但同样重要的是呼吁员工的利他主义，鼓励他们为社会、包括子孙后代做出贡献。

采取广泛的可持续性方法

采取广泛的可持续性做法十分重要，考虑以下几个方面：

- 能源和碳管理；
- 采购和食品；
- 旅行、运输和使用；

- *Water*;
- *Waste*;
- *The built environment*;
- *Organisational and workforce development*;
- *Partnership and networks*;
- *Governance*;
- *Finance*.

Imagine you are the director of a maternity service serving a deprived, multi-ethnic population. How would you recruit midwives? One approach is to advertise as widely as your budget allows with the aim of recruiting 'the best', but there are other approaches:

- *avoid depleting the midwifery workforces of poor countries as a matter of principle*;
- *develop a programme in which midwives visit local primary and secondary schools and encourage girls in the surrounding communities to consider midwifery as a career.*

Imagine you are a clinical director facing cuts to your budget. One approach is to reduce the costs of support services by outsourcing cleaning and secretarial services. This will reduce your financial costs but at the expense of the income of people who are already the lowest paid in the health service. Another approach is to establish stronger links with the surrounding communities, encouraging the recruitment of local people who are more likely to develop a commitment to the local service and fulfil their responsibilities assiduously irrespective of the level of their salary.

Local sourcing, and not outsourcing, can be applied to other aspects of running a health service. Clinicians could consider promoting the procurement of food from the local foodshed (usually defined as food grown or sourced within a 30-mile radius of the facility).

Apart from the environmental benefits of reducing "food miles" and thereby reducing carbon emissions, food sourced locally helps to retain money in the local economy and create wealth in the population served.

- 水；

- 废弃物；

- 建筑环境；

- 组织和劳动力发展；

- 合作关系和合作网络；

- 治理；

- 财政。

想象一下，你是一家为贫困、多民族人群服务的妇产医疗机构的主管。你将如何招聘助产士？一种方法是在预算允许的范围内尽可能广泛地发布广告，目的是招聘"最优人选"。但也有其他方法：

- 原则上避免从不发达国家招聘助产士；

- 制订一项计划，让助产士访问当地的中小学，并鼓励周围社区的女孩将助产士视为一种职业前景。

假设您是一名临床主任，面临削减预算。一种方法是通过外包清洁和秘书服务来降低后勤服务成本。这虽能减少经济成本，但却是以牺牲医疗卫生领域那些薪资最低者的收入为代价。另一种方法是与周围社区建立更牢固的联系，鼓励招募当地人，这些人更愿意在当地服务，兢兢业业地履行职责而不论其工资水平。

可以将本地采购（而不是外包）应用于医疗卫生运营的其他方面。临床医生可以考虑多从当地农产品商店采购食物［通常是指在该设施方圆30英里（约48千米）范围内种植或采购的食品］。除了通过减少"食物里程"来减少碳排放获得环境效益外，本地采购食物也有助于保留当地经济实力，并在所服务的人群中创造财富。

The realisation of sustainable development requires long-term planning, which takes into account not only the specific issues relating to healthcare facilities but also factors that could influence the determinants of health. Although addressing the health service's impact on the determinants of health requires a much wider scope than that currently taken by many people who manage healthcare, this type of approach is now recognised as necessary. As The Lancet Commission emphasised:

Sustainable development also 'includes notions of social justice and equity'. (22)

Equity is another key responsibility for the clinician practicing population medicine, and is discussed in Chapter 4.

■ Questions for reflection of for use in teaching or network building

If using these questions in network building or teaching, put one of the questions to the group and ask them to work in pairs to reflect on the question for three minutes; try to get people who do not know one another to work together. When taking feedback, let each pair make only one point. In the interests of equity, start with the pair on the left-hand side of the room for responses to the first question, then go to the pair on the right-hand side of the room for esponses to the second question.

- What steps can be taken to ensure that increases in productivity actually release cash?
- How can productivity and the need for greater productivity be explained on a local radio programme in 30 seconds?
- Do professionals have a duty to minimise cost?
- How could staff and patient travel be reduced in our service?
- How could we use less energy in heating and lighting in existing buildings, and how can we reduce future energy consumption in any plans for development of the healthcare estate?
- What scope do we have in our services for adopting the four principles of sustainable clinical practice?

实现可持续发展需要长期规划，不仅要考虑到与医疗卫生设施有关的具体问题，还要考虑对健康决定因素的影响。尽管解决医疗服务对健康决定因素的影响要远远超过医疗卫生管理人员目前的范围，但这种方法是必要的。正如柳叶刀委员会所强调的：

可持续发展亦包括社会公正和公平的概念。[22]

公平是临床医生实践群医学的另一项重要责任，第四章将对此进行讨论。

■ 互动思考题

如果在工作网络建设或教学中使用以下问题，可以将其中一个问题交给小组，让他们两人一组，思考3分钟，并尽量让彼此不认识的人一起工作。要求每组只能提出一个观点作为反馈。为了公平起见，让房间左侧的一组开始回答第1个问题，然后让房间右侧的一组开始回答第2个问题。

- 可以采取哪些措施来确保生产率提高的同时能够真正释放资金？
- 如何在30秒内通过本地广播节目解释生产力和提高生产力的必要性？
- 专业人士是否有责任将成本降至最低？
- 在我们的服务中，如何减少员工和患者的奔波？
- 我们如何减少现有建筑物的供暖和照明中能源的使用，以及如何在未来的医疗产业开发计划中减少能源消耗？
- 采用可持续临床实践四项原则的医疗卫生服务涉及哪些方面？

References

(1) Ohno, T.(1995) The Toyota Production System. Productivity Press.

(2) Black, J. and Miller, D.(2008) The Toyota Way to Healthcare Excellence. Increase Efficiency and Improve Quality with Lean. ACHE Management Series (p.236).

(3) Black, J. with Miller, D.(2008) The Toyota Way to Healthcare Excellence. Increase Efficiency and Improve Quality with Lean. ACHE Management Series.

(4) Toussaint, J., Gerard, R. and Womack, J.(2010) On the mend: revolutionizing healthcare to save lives and transform the industry.

(5) Berwick, D.M. and Hackbarth, A.D.(2012) Eliminating waste in US health care. Journal of the American Medical Association 307: 1513-1516.

(6) Chief Medical Officer for England (2005) Annual Report.

(7) Nelson, E.C., Batalden, P.B., Godfrey, M.M.(2007) quality by design. A clinical Microsystems Approach. John Wiley & Sons Inc.(p.7).

(8) Sibley, J.C. et al (1982) A randomized trial of continuing medical education NEJM 306; 511-515.

(9) Chalmers, I. and Glasziou, P.(2009) Avoidable waste in the production and reporting of research evidence. Lancet 374: 86-89.

(10) Gallacher, K., Montori V.M. and Mair, F.S.(2011) Understanding Patients' Experiences of Treatment Burden in Chronic Heart Failure Using Normalization Process Theory. Annals of Family Medicine 9: 235-243.

(11) Department of Health (2009) Equity and Excellence: Liberating the NHS.

(12) Claxton, K. et al.(2008) Value-based pricing for NHS drugs: an opportunity not to be missed. BMJ 336: 251-255.

(13) Brazier, J., Ratcliffe, J., Salomon, J.A. and Tsuchiya, A.(2007) Measuring and Valuing Health Benefits for Economic Evaluation. Oxford University Press.

(14) Mitton, C. and Donaldson, C.(2004) Priority setting toolkit. A guide to the use of economics in healthcare decision making. BMJ Publishing Group (p.47).

—— 参 考 文 献 ——

（15）Maslach, C. and Leither, M.P.（1997）The truth about burnout. San Francisco：Jossey-Bass. Cited in：Cole, T. R. and Carlin, N.（2009）The art of medicine：the suffering of physicians. Lancet 374：1414-1415.

（16）Brybye, L.N. and Shanafelt, T.D.（2011）Physician burnout：a Potential Threat to Successful Healthcare Reform. JAMA 305；2009-2010.

（17）Slim, W.（1956）Defeat Into Victory. Cooper Square Press.

（18）NHS Sustainable Development Unit（2009）Saving Carbon, Improving Health. NHS Carbon Reduction Strategy for England. January 2009.

http：//www.sdu.nhs.uk/documents/publications/1237308334_qylG_

（19）Connor, A. et al.（2010）The carbon footprint of a renal service in the United Kingdom. Quart. J.Med. 103：965-975.

（20）Middleton, J.（2008）Medicine, Conflict and Survival. Sandwell's Other Health Summit. 24, Supplement 1：S63

（21）Griffiths, J., Stewart, L.（2008）Sustaining a healthy future：taking action on climate change. The Faculty of Public Health,（p.12）.

（22）Lancet and University College London Institute for Global Health Commission.（2009）Managing the health effects of climate change. Lancet 373：1693-1733.（p.1719）.

（23）NHS Sustainable Development Unit（2010）Saving Carbon, Improving Health. Update. NHS Carbon Reduction Strategy.

http：//www.sdu.nhs.uk/publications-resources/42/NHS-Carbon-Reduction-Strategy-Update/

（24）Mortimer, F.（2010）The sustainable physician. Clinical medicine 10：110-111.

Chapter 4
MITIGATING INEQUITY

第四章
减少不公平

This chapter will:

- explain the difference between inequity and inequality;
- give examples of ways in which equity can be assessed;
- discuss the relationship of equity in healthcare to the broader issue of social justice.

By the end of the chapter, you will have developed an understanding of:

- how the concepts of equity and social justice are related;
- how to explain the term 'equity' and in what ways it differs from equality;
- how to explore the issue of equity, the Inverse Care Law and unmet need in your service.

■ Distinguishing inequity from inequality

Many people are confused about the difference between the terms 'inequality' and 'inequity', but the meaning of the two is quite different. Inequality is measured objectively; inequity is a subjective judgement of unfairness.

Health inequalities are measured and reported using criteria such as the standardised mortality ratio (SMR). In all countries, there is marked inequality among different social groups — the greater the level of deprivation the higher the mortality rate. This is clearly depicted in one of the classic visualisations of population health, the Jubilee Line map showing differences in male life-expectancy travelling east from Westminster — every two London Underground stops represent over one year of life-expectancy lost (see Figure 4.1).

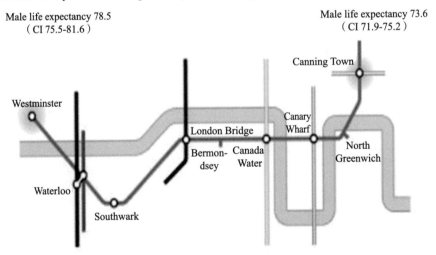

Figure 4.1 Differences in male life-expectancy within a small area of London

本章节涉及的内容：

- 解释不公平和不平等的区别；
- 举例说明评估公平的方法；
- 讨论医疗卫生公平与更广泛的社会公正问题的关系。

在本章末，读者将会深入理解：

- 公平与社会正义的概念是如何关联的；
- 如何解释"公平"这个词，它与"平等"的不同之处；
- 如何探讨公平、逆关怀法和未被满足医疗需求问题。

■ 区别不公平和不平等

许多人对"不平等（inequality）"和"不公平（inequity）"的区别感到困惑，但这两个词的含义确实有很大不同。不平等是客观衡量的；而不公平则是对不公平性（unfairness）的主观判断。

健康方面的不平等是以标准化死亡比（SMR）作为衡量和报告的指标。在所有国家，不同社会群体之间都存在明显的不平等：贫困程度越高，死亡率就越高。这一点在经典的人口健康可视化中得到了清晰的描述，伦敦地铁银禧线地图显示了从威斯敏斯特向东沿线的男性预期寿命的差异——每两个地铁站代表超过一年的预期寿命损失（图4.1）。

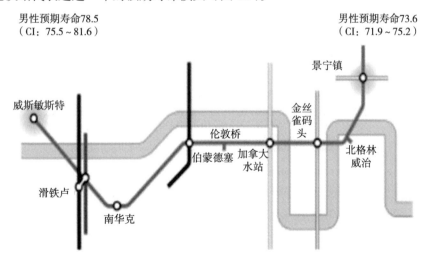

男性预期寿命78.5
（CI：75.5～81.6）

男性预期寿命73.6
（CI：71.9～75.2）

图4.1　伦敦某区域的男性预期寿命差异

The relationship between deprivation and ill-health is well documented, and the causal pathway linking the two is mediated through 'the social determinants of health', a term developed and popularized by Michael Marmot (1).

Inequalities in health service provision, however, do not follow the same pattern as inequalities in health. In both the Dartmouth Atlas of Health Care and the NHS Atlases of Variation in Healthcare, it is obvious that the distribution of many health services bears no consistent relationship to levels of deprivation in populations.

There can be marked variation for many aspects of health service provision among similarly wealthy populations and among similarly deprived populations. In the NHS Atlas of Variation in Healthcare for Children and Young People (2) and the NHS Atlas of Variation in Healthcare for Respiratory Disease (3), several indicators were used to investigate the variation among the 10 most-deprived populations and the 10 least deprived populations. As can be seen from Figure 4.2, the rate of admissions for bronchiolitis in children per 100, 000 population under two years (2008/09–2010/11) shows a 15-fold variation among the 10 most-deprived primary care trusts (PCTs) and a 2.7-fold variation among the 10 least-deprived PCTs.

It is vital that the clinician responsible for population medicine takes account of the health inequalities in the local population. This it is important because as part of a strategy to improve the health of the whole population it is necessary to try to reduce the level of health inequalities.

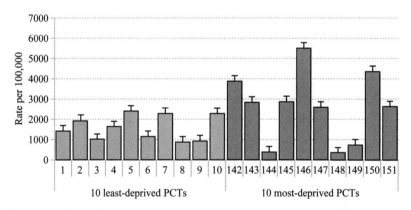

Figure 4.2 Rate of admissions for bronchiolitis in children per 100,000 population under two years; comparison of 10 least-deprived and 10 most-deprived primary care trusts (2008/09–2010/11). (2,3)

贫困与不健康之间的关系是由"健康问题的社会决定因素"来分析判断的，该术语由迈克尔·马尔莫特提出并推广[1]。

然而，医疗卫生保健供给方面的不平等与健康方面的不平等并不遵循同样的模式。在达特茅斯医疗卫生图集和NHS医疗卫生变化图集中，很明显，许多卫生资源的分布与人口的贫困程度没有一致性。

在同样富裕的人群和同样贫困的人群中，卫生服务提供的许多方面可能存在显著差异。在NHS儿童青少年医疗卫生变化图谱[2]和NHS呼吸系统疾病医疗卫生变化图谱[3]中，使用了几个指标来调查10个最贫困群体和10个贫困程度最轻的群体之间的差异。从图4.2可以看出，前10位最贫困的英国初级卫生保健信托机构（PCT）[1]之间每10万名2岁以下人口中的毛细支气管炎儿童入院率（2008年9月至2010年11月），存在15倍的差异，而前10名贫困程度最轻的PCT[1]之间存在2.7倍的差异。

负责群医学的临床医生必须考虑到当地人口的健康不平等。这一点很重要，因为作为改善全民健康战略的一部分，必须努力降低健康不平等的程度。

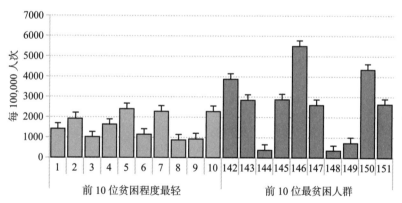

图4.2　前10位最贫困人群和贫困程度最轻前10位人群的比较（2008/09-2010/11）[2,3]；每10万人2岁以下儿童毛细支气管炎入院比例

① 译者注：英国初级卫生保健信托机构很大程度而言相当于管理机构，其职责是负责委托初级卫生保健、社区医疗和二级卫生保健服务，在2011年12月31日之前，英国初级卫生保健信托机构也直接提供社区医疗服务。按照2012年英国《健康和社会保障法案》，初级卫生保健信托机构于2013年3月31日废除，其原有职责由临床委托小组接管。临床委托小组由全科医生、护士和其他卫生专业人士组成，并受到当地的社工服务团队的支持。

In fact, recent cross-national evidence suggests that the greater the degree of socio-economic inequality that exists within a society, the steeper the gradient of health inequality. As a result, middle-income groups in a more unequal society will have worse health than comparable or even poorer groups in a society with greater equality. Of course, we cannot infer causation from correlation, but there are plausible hypotheses about pathways which link social inequalities to health, and, even if more work remains to be done to clarify the exact mechanisms, it is not unreasonable to talk here about the social 'determinants' of health. (4)

As mentioned at the beginning of this chapter, inequality is not the same as inequity. Thomas Rice, a highly respected economist, emphasizes the importance of distinguishing between the concepts of equality and equity:

The former implies equal shares of something; the latter, a 'fair 'or' just 'distribution, which may or may not result in equal shares. (5)

■ Classifying inequity in health services

There are several different types of inequity in the provision of health services (see Box 4.1).

Box 4.1 Types of inequity in the provision of health services

- Age-related, when older people are denied treatment simply because of their age
- Gender-related, when women receive effective treatment less frequently than men (10)
- Ethnicity-related, when members of a particular ethnic group receive less care than members of other ethnic groups despite the same level of or greater need as a result of either cultural insensitivity or racism (11、12)
- Social, when one socio-economic group, almost always the most deprived, does not have the same access to healthcare as other socio-economic groups

If there are lower rates of intervention in one subgroup of the population which has the same, or greater, need than the population as a whole, this would suggest there are problems with the equity of provision. If patients in one subgroup of the population receive treatment at a later stage in the course of the disease than patients in another subgroup, this would also suggest problems with the equity of

事实上，最近的多国证据表明，一个社会中存在的社会经济不平等程度越大，健康不平等的梯度就越大。因此，中等收入群体的健康状况在一个不平等程度较大的社会中，将比在一个相对平等的社会中的同等群体甚至更贫穷的群体更差。当然，我们无法从相关性中推断因果关系，但一些合理的假说可解释社会不平等与健康之间的联系，即使还需要做更多的工作来澄清确切的机制，我们也可以在这里谈论有关健康的社会"决定因素"。[4]

如本章开头所述，不平等并不等同于不公平。托马斯·赖斯这位备受尊敬的经济学家，强调要区分平等和公平概念的重要性：

前者意味着对某东西享有同等份额；后者意指在分配上要"公正（fair）"或"正义（just）"，但在份额上则可能"会"或"不一定会"同等。[5]

■ 医疗卫生保健服务不公平的分类

在医疗卫生保健服务的提供方面，有几种类型不同的不公平（专栏4.1）。

专栏4.1 在提供医疗卫生保健服务方面不公平的类型

- 与年龄相关的不公平：老年人仅因为年龄过大而被拒绝给予治疗。
- 与性别有关的不公平：女性接受有效治疗的频率低于男性[10]。
- 与种族有关的不公平：某一族群对医疗卫生保健服务需求水平与其他组群相差无异或更大，但由于文化钝感、种族主义或歧视，该族群成员得到的照顾少于其他族群的成员[11, 12]。
- 源于社会性的不公平：当某一社会经济群体（几乎总是最贫困的群体）得不到其他社会经济群体同样的医疗卫生保健服务。

当某一人群比总人群有更多的卫生需求时，但其得到的服务水平却低于总人群，这就意味着在供给的公平性上存在问题。如果相同疾病的患者仅因为所在的人群不同，便在疾病发展晚期才接受治疗，这也反映了在医疗供给供应的公平性方面存在问题。在英国进行髋关节和膝关节全置换的公平性研

provision. In a study of equity of access to total joint replacement of hip and knee in England, Judge et al. (6) concluded that people in affluent areas got most provision relative to need (see Figure 4.3).

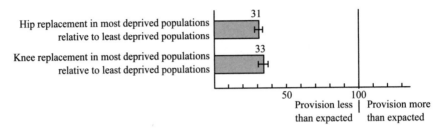

Figure 4.3 Inequities in the provision of hip and knee replacement (6)

It is also important to be aware that there can be situations in which inequality is equitable. For instance, a health service may decide to provide more resources to a deprived population because the need is greater than that in a less-deprived population.

Process equity should be the goal of health systems. There are several ways in which process equity can be defined.

- *Equal access to health care for equal need*
- *Equal use of health care for equal need*
- *Equal health care expenditure for equal need.*

All of these refer to equity between people with the same health care needs. This is known as horizontal equity. It is also important to recognize the corollary, that people with different or unequal needs should receive different or unequal health care. This is known as vertical equity. (7)

Another dimension to the concept of healthcare inequity relates to the quality of care provided and not just the volume of care or activity levels. In 1971, Julian Tudor Hart, an exceptional general practitioner, published an article describing the Inverse Care Law, which states that:

the availability of good medical care tends to vary inversely with the need for it in the population served. (8)

究中，贾琦（Judget）等人[6]得出的结论是，富裕地区的人们获得了最能满足需求的供给量（图4.3）。

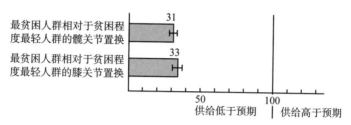

最贫困人群相对于贫困程
度最轻人群的髋关节置换 31

最贫困人群相对于贫困程
度最轻人群的膝关节置换 33

50   100

供给低于预期 | 供给高于预期

图4.3 在髋关节和膝关节置换手术方面存在的供给不公平

在某些情况下，不平等（inequality）是公平的（equitable）。认识到这点同样重要。例如，卫生服务机构可能会决定向贫困人群提供更多的资源，因为这些人的需求大于那些相对富裕的人群。

程序公平应该是卫生体系的目标。通过以下方法可以定义程序公平：

● 需求相同者有同等可及医疗卫生保健服务的机会；

● 需求相同者使用了同等医疗卫生保健服务；

● 为需求相同者支出了同等医疗费用。

所有这些都是指具有相同医疗卫生需求的人之间的公平。这就是所谓的横向公平。以此类推，需求不同或不平等的人在得到医疗卫生服务方面就也应该相应地不同或不平等。这就是所谓的纵向公平。[7]

医疗卫生不公平的另一个概念与其质量有关，而不仅只是服务的数量或频次。1971年，朱利安·都铎·哈特，一位杰出的全科医生，发表了一篇关于逆向照护法则的文章，文章指出：

在一个地区，高质量医疗卫生保健的可获得性往往与所服务人群的需求成反比。[8]

A clear illustration of the Inverse Care Law in operation is the experience of single homeless people whose needs are high but who, in most cities, have very poor access to care and therefore receive less high-value care.

■ Identifying inequity

Some of the root causes of inequity are outwith the power of the medical profession to solve, but the individual clinician with responsibility for a population can mitigate the effects of inequity by identifying people within the population who are likely to be experiencing inequity (see Box 4.2).

Box 4.2 Ways to identify inequity in the population being served

- Compared the number of patients seen from different subgroups within the population, e.g. from different general practices, social groups, or ethnic groups
- Audit referrals to identify differences in levels of need at the point of referral in different groups of patients

Having identified inequity, the clinician responsible for a population can take action by:

- *making a direct approach to the relevant subgroups in the population, such as engaging with a mosque or church in the locality;*
- *visiting health centres serving populations from which referrals seem too few.*

It is, however, difficult for any clinician to achieve much as an individual. It is important to persuade the healthcare organization to take action:

- *by including representatives of the most deprived subgroups in the population on boards and management groups;*
- *by investing in the local population, through establishing scholarships at local schools and colleges with the aim of recruiting more local people into the healthcare professions and workforce.*

单身流浪汉的经历清楚地说明了逆向照护法则是真实存在的。他们的卫生需求很高，但在大多数城市，他们的医疗卫生可及性很低，因此，得到高质量医疗卫生服务的机会较少。

■ 识别不公平

消除某些不公平的根源性因素非医学界力所能及，但负责人群健康的临床医生自己可以通过识别人群中可能遭遇不公平待遇的那些人，进而减轻不公平带来的影响（专栏4.2）。

专栏4.2　识别服务人群中存在不公平的方法

- 比较人群中来自不同亚人群的患者数量，如来自不同的全科门诊、社会群体或种族群体。
- 审核转诊，以确定不同患者人群在转诊时医疗需求水平的差异。

在识别出不公平之后，负责该人群的临床医生可以采取以下措施：

- 直接接触人群中的相关人群，例如与当地的清真寺或教堂接触；
- 访问那些转诊人数过少的医疗卫生服务中心。

然而，作为个体，任何临床医生都很难取得很大成就。因此，说服医疗卫生保健机构采取措施是很重要的：

- 将人口中最贫困人群的代表纳入管理委员会或管理小组；
- 通过向当地人群投资，在当地学校和大学设立奖学金，目的是吸引更多的当地年轻人加入医疗卫生保健服务行业。

■ Equity and social justice

It is important for the leadership of any healthcare organisation to appreciate the multidimensional nature of equity; as a concept, it cannot be understood solely in terms of the distribution of healthcare.

Health equity has many aspects, and is best seen as a multidimensional concept. It includes concerns about achievement of health and the capability to achieve good health, not just the distribution of health care. But it also includes the fairness of processes and thus must attach importance to non-discrimination in the delivery of health care. Furthermore, an adequate engagement with health equity also requires that the considerations of health be integrated with broader issues of social justice and overall equity, paying adequate attention to the versatility of resources and the diverse reach and impact of different social arrangements. (9)

Equity is a matter of social justice, and any publicly funded health service has a part to play in creating a just society as well as a healthy society; indeed, some would argue that a population cannot be healthy if there is significant injustice.

Justice...requires meeting health care needs fairly under resource constraints and this, in turn, requires limiting care in a publicly accountable way. (10)

Taking this perspective, health promotion encompasses efforts not only to change individuals' lifestyles but also to promote social justice.

■ Questions for reflection or for use in teaching or network building

If using these questions in network building or teaching, put one of the questions to the group and ask them to work in pairs to reflect on the question for three minutes; try to get people who do not know one another to work together.When taking feedback, let each pair make only one point.In the interests of equity, start with the pair on the left-hand side of the room for responses to the first question, then go to the pair on the right-hand side of the room for responses to the second question.

- What can be done by the NHS to tackle inequity in access to healthcare when the causes of inequity are so deeply embedded in society?

■ 公平和社会正义

任何医疗卫生保健组织的领导者都必须认识到公平的多维性；公平作为一个概念，不能仅从医疗卫生分配上来理解。

健康的公平有很多方面，最好能将其视为一个多维概念。它包括关注健康结果和实现健康的能力，而不仅是卫生服务的分布，同时它也包括程序公平，因此在提供医疗卫生保健时，必须重视非歧视原则。此外，充分处理健康公平问题，还需要把健康问题与社会公正和总体公平等更广泛的问题相结合；也要充分注意资源的灵活性以及不同社会安排的范围和多种影响。[9]

公平反映的是一种社会正义。任何公共资助的卫生服务都有助于创造一个健康和公正的社会。当然有些人还会争论说，如果存在严重的社会不公正现象，那么人群就不可能健康。

公正……需要在资源有限时公平地满足医疗卫生的需求。反过来，也需要以对公众负责的方式对医疗卫生保健服务的范围有所限制[10]。

从这个角度来看，健康促进不仅应包括改变个人生活方式的努力，还应致力于促进社会的公正。

■ 互动思考题

如果在工作网络建设或教学中使用以下问题，可以将其中一个问题交给小组，让他们两人一组，思考3分钟，并尽量让彼此不认识的人一起工作。要求每组只能提出一个观点作为反馈。为了公平起见，让房间左侧的一组开始回答第1个问题，然后让房间右侧的一组开始回答第2个问题。

- 当不平等的成因深深根植于社会之中时，NHS可以做些什么来解决医疗卫生方面的不公平问题？

- When considering your service, which subgroups in the local population are at greatest risk of inequity?
- What could you do next year to reduce inequity in your service?

References

(1) WHO (2008) Closing the gap in a generation: Health equity through action on the social determinants of health; report of the Commission chaired by Michael Marmot.

(2) Right Care (2012) NHS Atlas of Variation in Healthcare for Children and Young People. Reducing unwarranted variation to increase value and improve quality. March 2012. http: //www.rightcare.nhs.uk/atlas/

(3) Right Care (2012) NHS Atlas of Variation in Healthcare for People with Respiratory Disease. Reducing unwarranted variation to increase value and improve quality. September 2012. http: //www.rightcare.nhs.uk/atlas/

(4) Daniels, N., Kennedy, B. and Kawachi, I. (2004) Health and Inequality, or, Why Justice is Good for Our Health. In: Anand, S., Peter, F. and Sen, A. Public Health, Ethics, and Equity. Oxford University Press (p.63).

● 谈及您所提供的医疗卫生保健服务，当地人群中的哪一个亚人群可能面临最大的不公平风险？

● 在您的医疗卫生保健项目中，未来您打算用什么措施来减少其中的不公平？

参 考 文 献

（5）Rice, T.（1998）The Economics of Health Reconsidered. Health Administration Press（p.152）.

（6）Judge, A. et al.（2010）Equity in access to total joint replacement of hip and knee in England. Br. Med. J. doi 10/1136bmj. c4902.

（7）Wonderling, D., Gruen, R. and Black, N.（2005）Introduction to Health Economics. Understanding Public Health. Open University Press（p.157）.

（8）Hart, J.T.（1971）The Inverse Care Law. Lancet 392: 48-49.

（9）Sen, A.（2004）Why Health Equity?In: Anand, S., Peter, F. and Sen, A.（Eds）Public Health, Ethics, and Equity. Oxford University Press（p.31）.

（10）Daniels, N. and Sabin, J.（2008）Setting Limits Fairly. Learning to share resources for health. Second edition. Oxford University Press（p.13）.

Chapter 5
PROMOTING HEALTH AND PREVENTING DISEASE

第五章
促进健康和预防疾病

This chapter will:

- offer several definitions of health;
- describe the relationship between health equity and justice;
- explain the part that a clinician can play in disease prevention.

By the end of the chapter, you will have developed an understanding of:

- why every health service must play a part in disease prevention;
- how hospital health services can contribute to improving health;
- whether the clinician practising population medicine has a responsibility for advocacy on behalf of the population's health.

■ The meanings of 'health'

The meaning of the term 'health' is problematic and under continuous evolution. However, there is a general consensus that a health service in isolation cannot promote health and prevent disease because it has no operational jurisdiction over almost all of the social determinants of health. Although all clinicians have a responsibility to promote health and prevent disease by providing information and support to the individual patients who consult them, this responsibility is of equal or greater significance for the clinician practicing population medicine.

The well-known definition of health enshrined in the WHO Constitution of 1948 serves a useful function:

Health is a complete state of physical, mental and social wellbeing and not merely the absence of disease or infirmity. (1)

Some authorities, however, argue that this definition is too narrow. For Amartya Sen, the concept of health should encompass two other concepts:

- *social justice*;
- *the societal responsibility to ensure that every individual has the capability of achieving their full potential* (2).

本章节涉及的内容：

● 提出"健康"的多重定义；

● 阐述健康"公平"与"公正"的联系；

● 阐明临床医生在疾病预防中发挥的作用。

在本章末，读者将会深入理解：

● 为什么医疗卫生保健服务必须在疾病的预防中发挥作用；

● 医疗卫生保健服务如何促进人群健康；

● 从事群医学的临床医生是否有责任在群体的健康方面进行宣传倡导。

■ "健康"的含义

"健康"一词的含义一直存在争议并不断演变。然而，人们普遍认为，孤立的医疗卫生保健服务不能有效地促进健康并预防疾病，因为它对涉及健康的几乎所有社会决定因素都没有实际管辖权。尽管所有临床医生都有责任向前来咨询的患者提供信息和支持，帮助他们促进健康、预防疾病；但对于从事群医学的医生来说，这一职责具有同等或更大的意义。

1948年《世界卫生组织宪章》中所载的众所周知的、具有实用性的"健康"定义为：

健康是生理、心理和社会适应的完好状态，而不仅是没有疾病或身体虚弱。[1]

一些权威人士认为这一定义过于狭隘。阿马蒂亚·森就认为健康的概念还应包括以下两个的概念：

● 社会公正；

● 使所有人都能充分发挥其最大潜能社会责任[2]。

Other distinguished philosophers, notably Norman Daniels, argue that this type of very broad definition is not useful.

> *I shall follow Boorse's (1997) suggestion and say that health is the absence of pathology. (Admittedly, 'health is the absence of pathology' has neither the ring nor the familiarity of 'health is the absence of disease'.) We may understand 'pathology' to refer to any deviation from the natural functional organization of a typical member of a species...is a departure from normal functioning...*
>
> *Before saying more about understanding health as normal function, I want to forestall a common misunderstanding about the narrowness of this biomedical conception.*
>
> *The conceptual narrowness is required. Health is not all there is to well-being or happiness, contrary to the famous World Health Organization (WHO) definition: 'Health is a state of complete physical, mental, and social well-being, and not merely the absence of disease or infirmity.' The WHO definition risks turning all of social philosophy and social policy into health care. (3)*

If we focus on Daniels' definition of health, which is narrower than that of Sen, it becomes all the more apparent that health services whose primary function is the diagnosis and treatment of disease should be involved in promoting and protecting the health of the population they serve, especially when the definitions given below are used to guide health service activity.

- *Health promotion comprises efforts to enhance positive health and reduce the risk of ill-health. (4)*
- *Health protection comprises legal or fiscal controls, other regulations and policies, and voluntary codes of practice. (4)*

From Sen's perspective, health workers should be concerned about social injustice even if it does not cause disease or complicate treatment, whereas Daniels' definition means that health workers should focus on injustice and inequity only when they are complicating factors in the prevention or treatment of disease.

而其他杰出的哲学家，尤其是诺曼·丹尼尔斯，认为这种宽泛的定义并无实用价值。

"我赞同布尔斯（1997）的观点，健康指的是无病理性病变。（然而，"无病理性病变"与"无疾病才是健康"二者间既无提示作用，公众对前者也不熟悉。）我们可能理解"病理"指的是偏离某个物种本身的自然属性功能……即不具备正常的生理性功能……

在阐述更多关于健康的正常机体功能之前，我想先指出在生物医学的狭窄领域里，人们所共同存在的误解。

概念的范围需要缩小。健康未必全部是社会福祉或幸福感，而与世界卫生组织关于健康的定义有所不同。世界卫生组织的定义是：健康是生理、心理和社会适应的完好状态，而不仅是没有疾病或身体虚弱。世界卫生组织关于健康的定义的问题在于，这将所有社会哲学和社会政策的风险都转化到卫生服务上了。[3]

如果我们仔细思考丹尼尔斯对于健康的定义，会发现它比森的定义更狭义，尤其是用于医疗卫生服务相关活动时。它将医疗卫生服务的基本功能直接定义为诊断和治疗疾病，并在服务的对象人群中促进健康和预防疾病。

- 健康促进包含提高健康水平和降低疾病风险的所有努力。[4]
- 健康保护包含法律、经济调控、其他规章政策和公众自觉的行为。[4]

森认为，卫生工作者应该关注社会不公正，即使它不会引发疾病或使治疗复杂化。但丹尼尔斯则认为只有当不公正和不公平等因素影响到疾病的预防和治疗时，卫生工作者才应该关注它们。

■ The clinician's contribution

In some countries, public health professionals view public health as a medical specialty. In other countries, in addition to the organization of primary and secondary preventive services (e.g. smoking cessation and screening, respectively), public health professionals focus on environmental protection or interpret their role as one of advocacy for social change.

However, clinicians primarily involved in diagnosis, treatment and care can also have a very important role to play in disease prevention. Although the public health professional is trained in the effective delivery of preventive services, the clinician has charismatic authority. While a public health professional may have charismatic authority, it tends to carry less impact with the general public and partner organisations. For instance, a report by a well-respected public health professional will have less effect than a media interview with a doctor in a white coat or scrubs. The impact of a trainee surgeon speaking about knife wounds, an emergency room specialist testifying to the terrible consequences of binge drinking, and a lung specialist holding a cancerous lung in a bottle needs to be harnessed more often.

However, there are many less dramatic steps that can be taken by a clinician practising population medicine in order to prevent disease, for example, by ensuring that:

- *everyone with heart disease, and not just those referred, are receiving aspirin and other evidence-based measures to control risk factors for a recurrent heart attack;*
- *every person with chronic lung and heart disease is receiving flu immunisation;*
- *every individual with tuberculosis is supported during the course of therapy until they have been cured;*
- *all the relatives of people diagnosed with familial hypercholesterolaemia are identified and invited for testing.*

Preventive healthcare is the most sustainable type of healthcare, but it requires focus and coordination, not only by public health professionals but also by practitioners of population medicine. Although some hospitals are now appointing public health professionals, this does not reduce the need for clinicians to be responsible for, and take action to improve, the health of the whole population.

■临床医生的贡献

在一些国家，公共卫生专业人员将公共卫生视为一门医学专业；在另一些国家，除了组织实施初级和二级预防（如戒烟和筛查）服务，公共卫生专业人员还聚焦于环境保护，或视自身角色为社会变革的倡导者。

然而，主要从事诊断、治疗和照护工作的临床医生，在疾病预防方面也可以发挥非常重要的作用。尽管公共卫生专业人员在疾病预防方面接受过专业的训练，但对公众而言，临床医生更具有权威性。即使一个公共卫生专家很有权威，他对于公众及合作机构的影响力会很小。例如，即使具有较高权威的公共卫生专家在做报告时，其产生的影响力也低于穿白大褂或者手术衣的医生接受媒体时的采访讲话。而后者的影响力就好比外科实习医师介绍刀伤、急诊专科医师证明酗酒会产生严重后果、呼吸专科医师拿着瓶装肺癌标本，需要更经常地加以利用。

然而，为从事群医学的临床医生可以采用一些日常步骤来预防疾病，例如，"确保"：

- 每个心脏病患者，而不仅是转诊过来的患者，都接受阿司匹林和其他循证干预措施，以控制引起复发性心肌梗死的危险因素；
- 每个患有慢性肺病和心脏病的人都接种流感疫苗；
- 每个肺结核患者在治疗过程中都会得到支持，直至治愈；
- 要找到被诊断为家族性高胆固醇血症的人的所有亲属，并都进行胆固醇检测。

疾病预防是最具有可持续性的卫生服务工作，但它不仅需要公共卫生专业人员，也需要群医学实践者们的关注与合作。虽然现在一些医院任命公共卫生专业人员从事这方面工作，但临床医生需要为整体人群健康负责并为之采取行动，这方面的需求从未减少。

■ Authority, leadership and action

Clinicians with management responsibilities have bureaucratic authority within the institution at which they fulfil those responsibilities. Clinicians practising population medicine will have some bureaucratic authority, but to fulfil their responsibilities they will have to employ other forms of authority:

- *sapiential authority, derived from their knowledge*;
- *charismatic authority, derived from their leadership position.*

Management is a set of processes that can keep a complicated system of people and technology running smoothly. The most important aspects of management include planning, budgeting, organizing, staffing, controlling, and problem solving. Leadership is a set of processes that creates organizations in the first place or adapts them to significantly changing circumstances. Leadership defines what the future should look like, aligns people with that vision, and inspires them to make it happen despite the obstacles.(5)

Management is mainly a transactional process, whereas leadership should be transformational, and not simply transactional. Thus, a leader not only has to deliver results but also has to transform organisations that serve the population. Transformational leadership may require that a clinician responsible for population medicine tries to improve the prevention of disease through advocacy:

- *by visiting the local Member of Parliament (MP)*;
- *by seeking to influence directly national or international policymaking*;
- *by ensuring that the relevant professional organisation is fully engaged in debates and decisions that could reduce the risk of disease.*

As the line of accountability in population medicine is to the population served and not to the Chief Executive of a bureaucracy, the clinician practising population medicine may need to take action without seeking permission and should remember the old adage 'It is easier to seek forgiveness than permission'. For instance, it would be appropriate for a clinician to brief a local Member of Parliament on the need for alcohol legislation without first asking the Chief Executive's permission, but it would be inappropriate to criticize the organisation to which they belong unless they had attempted to achieve change in the first place before deciding to 'blow the whsitle'.

■ 权威、领导力和行动

具有管理职责的临床医生在履职机构中拥有行政权威。从事群医学的临床医生也拥有一些行政权威，但为了充分履职，他们还必须使用其他形式的权威：

- 源于知识的智慧权威；
- 来自领导地位的魅力权威。

管理是确保人员和技术的复杂系统顺利运行的一整套过程。管理最重要的职能包括计划、预算、组织、人员配置、控制以及解决问题。领导力是建立组织或使其适应变化环境的一整套过程。领导力描绘了未来的蓝图，使人们与这一愿景保持一致，并激励他们克服障碍，使之成为现实。[5]

管理主要是事务性的过程，而领导力应该具有变革性。因此，一个领导者不仅要取得成果，还必须变革为民众服务的组织。变革型领导力可能要求负责群医学的临床医生尝试以下方式以提高预防疾病的能力：

- 拜访当地政要；
- 试图直接影响国家或国际的政策制定；
- 确保相关专业机构有充分机会参加与减少人群疾病风险相关内容的讨论和决策。

由于群医学的责任主体是所服务的人群而不是官僚机构的行政长官，因此，从事群医学的临床医生可能需要在不寻求许可的情况下采取行动，并应记住"寻求原谅比寻求许可更容易"这句老话。例如，临床医生可以不首先征求行政长官的同意，而向当地议员介绍酒精立法的必要性。但批评自身所属的组织却是不妥的，除非他们在决定"吹哨"之前已打算改弦易辙、急于变革。

■ Hospitals as health services

Language creates the culture within which people make decisions and express various behaviours. The traditional bureaucratic division of health services and the language used to describe these services — 'hospital' and 'community' in relation to care and the separate identification of 'mental health services' — creates the wrong culture, one in which the hospital is assumed to be outside the community and only in the healthcare and not the health business (see Figure 5.1). Hospital services, however, can play a major role in improving the health of the populations they serve, and acting as a public health service.

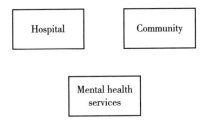

Figure 5.1 Healthcare as an archipelago

'Public health' is another term that causes confusion because it is, in one sense, a description of a professional group, in another the outcome of the efforts of everyone seeking to prevent, diagnose and treat disease and promote health. Some hospitals are now setting up public health departments which have public health professionals within them, an approach sometimes called 'the health-promoting hospital'. These departments sometimes focus on ensuring that every person who comes into hospital as a patient receives help to stop smoking. Although such moves are welcome, it is important not to create the impression that it absolves every other department in the hospital from using their opportunities and influence to promote health and prevent disease. Every hospital department has the ability to influence the health of the population served:

- *the trauma team can campaign against knife crime;*
- *the hepatology service can campaign against harmful and hazardous drinking;*
- *the cardiology service can promote exercise and physical activity.*

■ 医院作为卫生服务机构

语言创造了文化，人们在其中做出决策、展示不同行为。卫生服务机构在传统行政划分以及用来描述这些机构的语言——如与医疗卫生相关的"医院"和"社区"以及对"精神卫生机构"的单独划分——形成了错误的文化；其中之一是认为"医院"应该设在社区之外，它只在卫生服务范畴之内行事，而不属于卫生事业（图5.1）。然而，医院服务可以在改善其服务人群的健康方面发挥主要作用，亦能履行公共卫生职能。

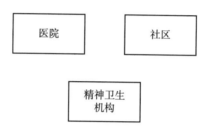

图5.1 医疗卫生保健"群岛"

"公共卫生"是另一个引起混淆的术语，因为在某种意义上，它是对一个卫生专业队伍的描述；从另一种意义上来说，它是每个人在预防、诊断和治疗疾病及健康促进方面所付出努力的结果。现在一些医院设立了公共卫生科室，其中雇有公共卫生专业人员，并被称为"健康促进医院"。这些科室有时会把工作重点放在帮助那些求助戒烟的就诊者。尽管此举受到了欢迎，但重要的是不要给人留下这样的印象，即医院的其他部门就没有责任利用机会和影响力以促进健康并预防疾病。医院的每个科室都有能力影响其服务整体人群的健康水平：

● 创伤救治小组可以呼吁打击持刀犯罪；

● 肝病服务中心可以开展反对有害饮酒的运动；

● 心脏病服务中心可以开展促进身体活动。

In addition, the hospital as a whole can contribute to improving the health of the population it serves. For instance, in South Auckland, the Middlemore Hospital decided not to recruit more nurses and health workers from the Philippines or Thailand but instead set up a Health Academy to inspire young people from the Maori and Pasifika communities to aspire to become health workers at Middlemore with great success.

■ Questions for reflection or for use in teaching or network building

If using these questions in network building or teaching, put one of the questions to the group and ask them to work in pairs to reflect on the question for three minutes; try to get people who do not know one another to work together. When taking feedback, let each pair make only one point. In the interests of equity, start with the pair on the left-hand side of the room for responses to the first question, then go to the pair on the righthand side of the room for responses to the second question.

- What is the most useful definition of health for a clinical service?
- How could a musculo-skeletal or mental health service contribute to the prevention of disease?
- What are the advocacy responsibilities of clinician practising population medicine?
- In what ways could a clinician ensure that locally and nationally elected representatives are adequately informed on population health issues?

References

(1) World Health Organization (WHO) Preamble to the Constitution of the World Health Organization as adopted by the International Health Conference, New York, 19 June-22 July 1946; signed on 22 July 1946 by the representatives of 61 States (Official Records of the World Health Organization, no.2, p.100) and entered into force on 7 April 1948. http: //www.who.int/suggestions/faq/en/index.html

(2) Sen, A.(2004) Why Health Equity?In: Anand, S., Peter, F. and Sen, A.(Eds) Public Health, Ethics, and Equity. Oxford University Press.

此外，医院可以作为一个整体为改善人群健康状况做出贡献。例如，在南奥克兰，米德莫尔医院决定不从菲律宾或泰国招聘更多的护士和卫生工作者，而是建立一所卫生学校，激励来自Maori和Pacific社区的年轻人成为米德莫尔医院的医疗卫生工作者，这项行动获得了极大的成功。

■ 互动思考题

如果在工作网络建设或教学中使用以下问题，可以将其中一个问题交给小组，让他们两人一组，思考3分钟，并尽量让彼此不认识的人一起工作。要求每组只能提出一个观点作为反馈。为了公平起见，让房间左侧的一组开始回答第1个问题，然后让房间右侧的一组开始回答第2个问题。

- 对一项临床服务而言，什么是对健康的最实用的定义？
- 在肌肉骨骼或心理健康领域的服务中，应当如何为预防疾病做出贡献？
- 践行群医学的临床医生，在宣传倡导方面应担负什么责任？
- 通过何种方式，临床医生可以保证其所在地区或国家所选的代表能充分理解人群健康的相关问题。

───── 参 考 文 献 ─

（3）Daniels, N.（2008）Just Health. Meeting health needs fairly. Cambridge University Press.

（4）Downie, R.S., Tannahill, C. and Tannahill, A.（1996）Health Promotion. Models and Values. Second edition. Oxford University Press.

（5）Kotter, J.（1996）Leading Change. Harvard Business School Press.

Chapter 6
DESIGNING POPULATION-BASED INTEGRATED SYSTEMS

第六章
设计以人群为基础的整合型体系

This chapter will:

- explain the difference between a system and an institution;
- define the basic components of a system, including the aim and objectives;
- describe each component of a system using examples as relevant;
- distinguish between individual outcomes and population outcomes.

By the end of this chapter, you will have developed an understanding of:

- the way in which the objectives for a system differ from the aim of a system;
- the way in which objectives can be set;
- the different types of criteria or measures that can be used to assess progress towards meeting the objectives;
- the way in which standards for a system can be set;
- The 20th century was the century of the institution; the 21st century is the century of the system.

■ From great institutions to great systems

In the Middle Ages, people built cathedrals; in the 19th century, they built railway stations; in the 20th century, they built hospitals. These hospitals became the great institutions of the 20th century, and the powerful and wealthy became members of hospital boards, similar to the way in which they had supported the Church in an earlier era, although few hospitals can hold a candle to the architectural glories of Notre Dame in Paris or St Pancras Station in London. Many hospitals are huge, sprawling sites, continually evolving and never reachingcompletion, like Sagrada Familia.

Hospitals became the sites for the delivery of specialist services, and also sites for the development of super-specialist services; these services came to be called secondary and tertiary care, respectively.

In addition, mental health services developed in the 19th century, most obviously in the form of asylums located on the edge of towns and cities remote from the hospitals, even though many of the residents had physical as well as mental problems, as is the case today.

In the second half of the 20th century, two new institutions developed-general practice and government-run community services. General practice evolved from be-

本章涉及内容：

- 解释体系和机构之间的区别；
- 定义体系的基本组成，包括目的和具体目标；
- 举例介绍体系的每个组成部分；
- 区分个体结果和群体结果。

在本章末，读者将会深入理解：

- 体系目标与目的区别；
- 目标的设定方式；
- 用于评估目标进展的不同类型的标准或指标；
- 设置体系标准的方式；
- 20世纪是机构的世纪，21世纪是体系的世纪。

■ 从大机构到大系统

中世纪的人们建造大教堂；19世纪的人们建造火车站；20世纪的人们则忙着建造医院。这些医院成为20世纪的伟大机构，权贵富人成为医院董事会的成员，类似于他们早期支持教会的方式，尽管很少有医院能与巴黎圣母院或伦敦圣潘克拉斯站的辉煌相提并论。许多医院都是杂乱无章的庞然大物，不断扩张，从未竣工，如圣家族大教堂。

医院成为提供专科医疗的场所，亚专科也在此处蜕变而出——这分别被称为二级和三级医疗。

此外，19世纪发展起来的精神卫生服务通常以收容所的形式运行，并且远离医院，位于城镇边缘，尽管很多精神病患者同时也有躯体上的疾患。时至今日，依然如此。

20世纪后半叶出现了两类新型机构——全科诊疗机构和政府运行的社区卫生服务机构。全科医生队伍由私营诊所中的一个个独立执业医生组成，随着皇家学院的建立和循证医学的发展，逐渐发展壮大。全科医生的兴起，部分是

ing composed of isolated practitioners in private practice to becoming a powerful force with the establishment of a Royal College and the development of an evidence base, in part as a consequence of the funding provided by the NHS. Community services provided voluntary and charitable services that had cared for the elderly, the infirm and children. The situation now, not only in the United Kingdom, is that healthcare is an archipelago with four great islands connected by the occasional ferry (Figure 6.1).

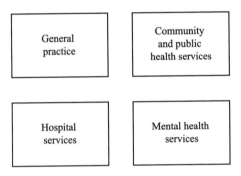

Figure 6.1 The healthcare archipelago

By the end of the 20th century there was also growing concern about the need to develop an integrated approach to common health problems through defining systems of care (1). The exemplar of an integrated system of care is that for people with cancer. Faced with the considerable capital expense of providing radiotherapy, the managers of most district general hospitals accepted that investment in that intervention should take place in teaching hospitals. This intensity of investment at some but not all healthcare site led to the creation of cancer networks, across which were delivered a system of care ranging from screening to end-of-life care. Constraints on capital investment also led to the development of systems for:

- *end-stage renal failure*;
- *acute stroke*;
- *myocardial infarction.*

In a population-based system, the archipelago of care is transformed into a set of inter-related types of care which recognises that self-care is the most important (Figure 6.2).

NHS提供资金的结果。而社区服务机构则为年老体弱者和儿童提供志愿和慈善服务。现在的情况是，不仅在英国，很多国家医疗卫生体系是由4个"孤岛"组成的，四大岛通过"临时渡轮"①相连（图6.1）。

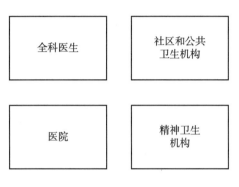

图6.1　医疗卫生体系"群岛"

到20世纪末，业界愈发达成共识需要通过定义医疗卫生体系，建立整合型体系以应对普遍存在的健康问题[1]。一个整合型卫生体系的范例是为癌症患者提供的医疗卫生服务。由于提供放射治疗需要大量资金支持，大多数地区综合医院的管理者都认为应仅为教学医院提供放疗资金。这种投资策略，即资金向少数医疗机构集中而非覆盖所有，促成了癌症工作网络的建立。通过该网络，为患者提供从筛查到临终关怀的一系列服务。与癌症同理，资金投入的限制也促成了以下疾病体系的发展：

- 终末期肾衰竭；
- 急性脑卒中；
- 心肌梗死。

在一个基于人群的体系中，医疗卫生保健服务"群岛"会被转型为彼此密切关联的各种医疗服务，并把患者的自我保健作为最重要的内容（图6.2）。

---

① 译者注：即转诊服务。

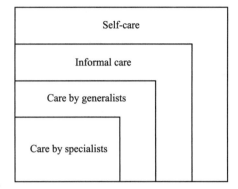

Figure 6.2 Four-box healthcare

Each system of care needs to have a focus. The various types of system focus for health services in countries with developed economies are shown in Box 6.1.

Box 6.1 The various types of focus for systems of care

- Symptoms or clinical presentations, such as breathlessness or back pain
- Diseases or conditions, such as inflammatory bowel disease, asthma or depression
- Subgroups of the population, such as frail elderly people or people under the 65 years of age with multiple morbidities

There can be tension between generalists and specialists but it is possible to minimise any tension by being clear about the relationship between complex and complicated health problems.

When discussing a condition such as asthma or epilepsy, it is common for general practitioners to point out that many of their patients have more than one problem. Indeed, people with multiple morbidities, often physical, mental and social, have complex problems — for example, an 84-year-old woman with four diagnoses and seven prescriptions being supported by a 50-year-old daughter with depression and a husband with an alcohol abuse problem. This is a complex problem but it is common in general practice. However, when one of the older woman's four problems, heart failure, for example, becomes complicated, the generalist needs to seek specialist advice. This highlights the relationship between complex and complicated problems, between the roles of generalist and specialist.

By contrast, in low-and middle-income countries, there is a move to create integrated primary care due to the inefficiencies that result from a collection of dis-

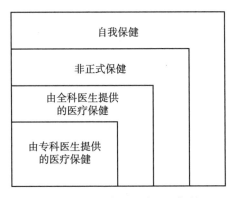

图6.2 "四层式"医疗卫生保健

每层医疗卫生体系都需要有一个关注点。专栏6.1展示了发达国家医疗卫生体系中不同类型的关注点。

专栏6.1 医疗卫生体系中不同类型的关注点

- 症状或临床表现，如呼吸困难或背痛；
- 疾病或患病状况，如炎性肠病、哮喘或抑郁症；
- 人群中的亚人群，如年老体弱者或65岁以下有多种疾病的人。

全科医生和专科医生之间的关系可能会因为分歧变得紧张，但双方如果能清楚地了解健康问题的复合性（complex）和病情的复杂性（complicated）之间的关系，紧张关系就可以大大缓解。

当讨论哮喘或癫痫等疾病时，全科医生通常会指出，许多患者的问题都不止一种。事实上，患有多种障碍（常为生理、心理和社会方面等问题）的人，都有复合性问题——例如，一位患有4种确诊疾病、接受7种处方治疗的84岁妇女，正由50岁患有抑郁症且丈夫酗酒的女儿赡养，这就是诊疗中常见的复合性问题。当这位老年妇女的4种疾病之一（如心力衰竭）变得复杂时，全科医生需要寻求专科医生的建议。这强调了疾病的复合性和复杂性之间的关系，以及全科医生和专科医生之间的关联。

相比之下，在低收入和中等收入国家，基于病种的（如盘尾丝虫病或疟疾）的医疗卫生体系各自为政、效率低下，这些国家正在探索建立整合型初

ease-based systems, such as onchocerciasis or malaria, which operate in isolation.

The development of systems of care does not reduce the need for good management of healthcare institutions, but it does require the skill to create and manage what have been called hybrid organisations, defined as organisations in which:

...functional units and mission orientated units work together and the accompanying principle of dual reporting, like a democracy, are not great in and of themselves. They just happen to be the best way for any business to be organised. (2)

Other people call this arrangement 'matrix management' and the pattern is emerging in many countries (see Matrix 6.1).

Matrix 6.1

		SYSTEMS					
		Cancer	Respiratory	Mental Health	Stroke	Frail Eilderly	Children
FACLITIES	HR						
	Transport						
	Finance						
	Real Estate						
	IT						

Andy Grove, who developed the definition of a hybrid organisation, was the Chief Executive of Intel and could control both dimensions of the matrix. The situation is more complex in healthcare where the contributions of different autonomous organisations must be integrated. This challenge requires the development of networks which will be discussed in Chapter 7.

■ The definition and design of a system

A system is a set of activities with a common set of objectives. To expand this definition, a system is a set of activities with a common aim and set of objectives, which produces an annual report for the population served, using criteria and standards common to all systems with the same focus.

The design and development of systems of care is described in detail in the companion book *How to Build Healthcare Systems*. The principal points in that book have been summarised in this chapter but some different examples have been used so the reader of this text will find new material. The design of a system has

级医疗卫生体系。

医疗卫生体系的发展不仅要求医疗卫生机构能够一如既往地良性管理，而且要求其具备建立和管理混合型组织的技能，即：

……一般职能部门和专业职能部门共事，以及随之而来的双重报告原则，就像民主制度，其自身及内在并不优越，但在组织任何事务时它们却正好是最佳方式。[2]

这种布局被称为"矩阵式管理"，此模式正出现在许多国家中（矩阵6.1）。

矩阵6.1 矩阵式管理

		系统					
		癌症	呼吸道疾病	精神卫生	脑卒中	老年保健	儿童保健
机构	人力资源						
	运输						
	财政						
	不动产						
	信息技术						

英特尔的首席执行官安迪·葛洛夫提出了混合型组织的概念，可控制矩阵的两个维度。在医疗卫生领域，情况更为复杂：必须整合不同自治组织，使其在系统中所发挥作用。这一挑战需要开发工作网络，我们将在第7章中讨论。

■ 体系的定义和设计

体系是具有共同目标的一组活动的集合，可进一步扩展为：一个体系是具有共同目的的一组活动和一系列目标所组成。它们运用那些对一切体系都通用的共同指标和标准，围绕着共同的核心内容，向所服务人群提供年度报告。

卫生体系的设计和开发在配套书籍《如何构建医疗卫生体系》中进行了详细描述。本章总结了该书中的主要观点，但使用了一些不同的示例，因此

several stages (see Box 6.2). For the rest of this chapter, the first five stages of designing and developing a system will be described, including the practical steps that can be taken at each stage. To accomplish the first five stages in the process, it will require several meetings of the team responsible for system development, at least five meetings of various stakeholders who will be involved in delivering the system of care under development, and time for wider consultation between stakeholder meetings.

Box 6.2 Stages in the design of a system of care

- Define the scope of the system
- Define the population for which the system has responsibility
- Reach agreement on the aim and objectives for the system
- For each objective, select one or more criteria with which to measure progress
- For each objective, set standards to enable benchmarking and comparison among services
- Reach agreement on the network of organisations necessary to deliver and govern the system (see Chapter 7)
- Identify the resources necessary to create a budget for the system (see Chapter 9)

The team responsible for system development should have representation from all the key organisations, and consultation should include other people who will be important in making sure the design is implemented. All the organisations and people involved in implementation comprise the network.

■ Defining the scope of the system

It is important to be aware that people may express in an unfocussed way and terms such as 'frail elderly' are used frequently without ever being clarified and agreed. To define the scope of a system, it is essential to identify the set of activities that need to be coordinated through the system. The scope should be as wide as is necessary to include every activity relevant to the aim. The team leading the development of the system are responsible for facilitating agreement on the activities to be included in the scope. Part of this facilitation process could involve testing or clarifying the boundaries of the scope through posing a series of questions (see Table 6.1).

本书的读者将读到新的内容。体系设计有几个步骤（专栏6.2）。在本章的其余部分，将描述体系设计和开发的前5个阶段，包括在每个阶段要采取的实际步骤。为了完成该过程的前5个阶段，需要召开几次负责体系开发的团队会议，包括至少5次是参与体系运行过程的利益攸关方的会议，也需要利益攸关方在每次会议中进行更广泛的协商。

专栏6.2　医疗卫生服务体系设计的各阶段

- 界定体系范围；
- 界定体系所服务的目标人群；
- 就体系的目的和目标达成共识；
- 就每项具体目标，选择一个或多个指标以测量其进展；
- 就每项目标设定衡量标准，以确保各项服务内容可通过基准进行比较；
- 在实施和管理体系时，应就各种机构的网络架构达成共识（见第7章）；
- 确定该体系所需资源的预算（见第9章）。

负责开发体系的团队应该包括所有关键机构的代表。要与其他重要人员进行磋商确保所设计的体系得以实施，由实施涉及的所有组织和人员组成"工作网络"。

■ 界定体系范围

我们需要意识到，人们表达的方式可能模糊不清，还有些术语如"年老体弱者"被频繁地使用，但含义却从未被界定清楚或取得共识。为了界定体系的范围，必须明确需要通过该体系进行协调的一系列活动。该范围应该尽量广泛，把所有与目标相关的必要活动都纳入其中。领导体系开发的团队负责协调各方，对需纳入服务范围的一系列活动达成共识。可以通过提出一系列问题来测试或澄清范围从而在一定程度上加快这一过程（表6.1）。

Table 6.1 Questions to clarify the scope of a system in relation to the system focus

System focus	Questions to clarify scope boundaries
Frail elderly people	● Should we use an arbitrary indicator such as being on four medications? ● Should we simply include everyone in a nursing home? ● Should we use a predictive risk score? ● Should we include everyone with dementia? ● Does it include end-of-life care?
Children	● Should we included neonates or should they be included in the scope for the maternity system? ● What is the upper age limit for children to be covered by the system? ● Is it better to establish a linked system for young people in transition, perhaps for those aged 15-24 years?
Musculo-skeletal programme	● Are people with fractures included in this system? ● Should there be a separate sub-system for people requiring joint replacement?

It is usually better to start with a subgroup of the population such as 'people at the end of life', rather than a service such as 'palliative care'. Using this approach, the real issue can be identified. For example, a discussion intended to develop an urgent care system quickly evolved into a focus on people with multiple morbidities, including both elderly (the 'frail elderly'), and people under 65 years who have considerable mental health and substance abuse problems. Sometimes a Venn diagram is more useful than a list (Figure 6.3).

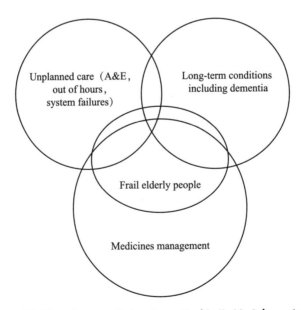

Figure 6.3 The subgroups that make up the 'frail elderly' population

表6.1 针对体系不同关注点来阐明其范畴的相关问题

体系关注点	阐明范畴的问题
年老体弱者	● 我们是否应该随意使用指标，例如在使用4种药物？ ● 我们是否应该简单地囊括每个在疗养院的人？ ● 我们应该使用预测风险评分吗？ ● 我们应该包括所有患有痴呆症的人吗？ ● 它包括临终关怀吗？
儿童	● 新生儿是否应该包括在内？还是应该将他们包括在产科体系范围内？ ● 该体系所涵盖的儿童年龄上限是多少？ ● 是否应该为转型期的年轻人，例如15～24岁建立一个连接体系？
肌肉-骨骼系统	● 该体系是否包括骨折患者？ ● 对于需要关节置换的人，是否应该有一个单独的子系统？

通常情况下，从界定一个对象群体的亚人群（处在生命末期的人群）入手以开启讨论，而不是以"舒缓医疗"之类的服务内容为入手来开始讨论，其效果更好。使用这种方法能确定真正的问题所在。例如，旨在发展急救医疗卫生照护体系的讨论可以迅速演变成针对患有多种疾病人群的讨论，涉及老年人群（年老体弱者）和65岁以下有严重精神健康问题和药物滥用问题的群体。在这些案例中，制作一张维恩图有时比列表更有用（图6.3）。

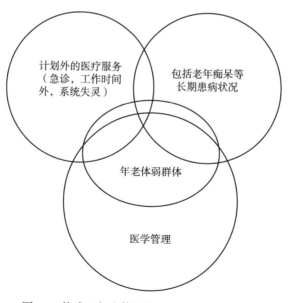

图6.3 构成"年老体弱者"人群的各种亚人群

Having defined the scope of the system, the next step is to define the population to be served.

■ Defining the population to be served

Each system of care has responsibility for a defined population. However, it is not always clear what should constitute the defined population for a particular system. For instance, although a population may appear to be clearly defined by a political jurisdiction such as a local authority, it is essential to define the population boundaries for a system of care because clinical communities of practice do not often correspond to politically defined jurisdictions. One way to define the population served by a system of care in the NHS is to 'construct' it from the relevant general practice populations given that general practices are responsible for the small populations that constitute the larger population. In countries in which insurance schemes ensure population coverage, the members of the scheme becomes the population.

At this stage, it is important to decide upon the optimum size of the population to be served by the system. In the traditional model of institution-based care, the size of the population served is about 300,000 people, based on the catchment population for a general hospital. The optimum population size for a system of care, however, is a function of several inter-related variables:

1. the incidence and prevalence of the problem — the size of the population must be large enough to include the number of clinical events sufficient to enable clinical expertise to be developed and for the production of a meaningful annual report;

2. the level of population need for super-specialist services and technology, such as neurosurgery.

The implications of two of these variables for optimum population size in relation to several different systems of care are shown in Table 6.2.

界定了该体系的范围，下一步就要界定目标人群。

■ 界定目标人群

每个医疗服务体系均有其特定的目标人群。然而，界定特定体系的人群构成通常比较困难。例如，虽然可能通过行政辖区（如地方当局）来明确人群的定义，但在临床实践的社区通常不等同于行政管辖区，因此必须为卫生体系定义人群的边界。界定 NHS 目标人群的方法之一，是根据相关全科医生服务的人群来"构建"，因为全科医生往往负责较大人群中的部分人群。在保险体系完善的国家，保险计划的成员可作为体系覆盖的人群。

在这一步中，重要的是要确定该体系能够服务人群的最佳规模。在基于医疗卫生机构的传统医疗服务模式中，服务人群的规模约为30万，这是基于一个综合医院所能覆盖的地理人群而言。然而，一个医疗服务体系的最佳服务人群规模取决于以下相互关联的因素：

1. 某种健康问题的发病率和患病率——人群规模必须大到包括足够的临床事件数量，以便发展临床专业技术并编撰有意义的年度报告；

2. 人群对诸如神经外科的亚专科的医疗和技术的需要的水平。

这两个变量可用于确定几个不同医疗服务体系的最佳人群规模，详见表6.2。

Table 6.2 The optimum size of population for a system

System focus	Incidence and prevalence	Population need for super-specialist intervention	Optimum population size
Asthma	High	Low	200,000-500,000
Epilepsy	High	High	There may need to be both a local support service for a smaller population—300,000—and a neurosurgical service related to a larger population—1 or 2 million—so that the local service's referral rates can be compared
Parkinson's disease	High	Low	300,000—500,000, although the need for deep brain stimulation may require a larger population size
Frail elderly people	High	Low	200,000-500,000
Motor neurone disease	Low	High	Support for this uncommon condition requires specialist teams

■ Reaching agreement on the aim and objectives

Aim: A high-level statement of the role of the department. (3)

Every system of care should have a single high-level aim with which all professionals and patients can identify. Examples of high-level aims are shown in Display 6.1.

Display 6.1 Examples of aims

Organisation	Aim
NASA	To put a man on the moon and bring him safely back (12 words)
National Breast Cancer Screening Programme	To offer women the opportunity of reducing their risk of dying from breast cancer (14 words)
A hospital	To offer high-quality, safe care tailored to meet the needs of each individual (13 words)

However, the aim of a system has to be complemented by a set of more detailed objectives on which everyone involved in providing care can focus their activities.

表6.2　每个体系关注点中的最佳人群规模

体系的关注点	发病率和患病率	人群对特殊亚专科的需求	最佳人群规模
哮喘	高	低	20万～50万人
癫痫	高	高	可能需要同时能针对较小人群的地方性支持服务（30万人）和对相对较大人群的神经外科服务（100万或200万人），这样就能对各个地方性服务的转诊率进行比较
帕金森病	高	低	30万～50万人，尽管行脑深部刺激治疗可能需要更大的人群规模
年老体弱者	高	低	20万～50万人
运动神经元病	低	高	需要有专家团队对这种罕见病提供技术支持

■ 就目的和具体目标达成共识

目的：是对部门使命的宏观阐述。[3]

每个医疗服务体系都应有能被所有医疗专业人员和患者识别的单一的宏观目的。场景6.1展示了高水准单一目的的一些例子。

场景6.1　目的范例

机构	目的
美国国家航空航天局	把一人送到月球并安全载回（12个英文单词）
国家乳腺癌筛查项目	降低妇女的乳腺癌死亡风险（14个英文单词）
一家医院	为每位患者提供"量身定制"、能满足其需要的、高质量的、安全的医疗服务（13个英文单词）

然而，一个体系的目的必须辅之以一系列更详细的目标，每个参与医疗的人都可以将他们的活动集中在这些目标上。

Objectives are needed in every area where performance and results directly and vitally affect the survival and prosperity of the business. ...Objectives should enable us to do five things:

- *to organize and explain the whole range of business phenomena in a small number of general statements;*
- *to test these statements in actual experience;*
- *to predict behaviour;*
- *to appraise the soundness of decisions when they are still being made; and*
- *to enable practising businessmen to analyse their own experience and, as a result, improve their performance.*

A draft set of objectives for a system for liver disease developed in a workshop is set out in Box 6.3.

Box 6.3 Draft set of objectives for a Liver Disease Programme

- To diagnose and treat liver disease quickly and accurately
- To treat liver disease effectively and safely
- To engage people with the condition and their carers as equal partners
- To promote the health of people with liver disease
- To develop the professionals who support people with liver disease
- To make the best use of resources
- To promote and support research
- To produce an annual report for the population served

There are two main types of objectives for a system of care:

1. 'clinical' objectives, which are analogues of traditional clinical activity, such as to diagnose accurately and quickly;

2. population objectives, relating to the use of resources for the whole population; population objectives are often overlooked by clinicians when setting the objectives for a system.

Practical steps involved in the development of a high-level aim for a system of care are shown in Box 6.4, and the practical steps involved in reaching agreement on the objectives for that system are shown in Box 6.5. At the same meeting, the group responsible for system development should also draft and agree a set of objectives. During the process of objective-setting, the scope may need to be

目标在任何领域对评价绩效、结果都是必需的，而且对事业的发展和繁荣至关重要……设立的目标应能使我们做以下五件事：

- 用简洁通俗的表述来描述和解释事情的全貌；

- 在实践中检验这些表述；

- 预测行为；

- 在做出决策时评估其合理性；

- 使执业者能够分析自己的经历，并据此提高绩效。

专栏6.3列举了草拟针对肝病服务项目的目标。

专栏6.3 草拟针对肝病服务项目的目标

- 快速、准确地诊断和治疗肝病。
- 有效、安全地治疗肝病。
- 在患者及其医疗卫生人员之间建立平等的伙伴关系。
- 改善肝病患者群体的健康状况。
- 培养为肝病患者提供支持的专业人员。
- 善用各种资源。
- 促进并支持研究工作。
- 向服务人群提供年度报告。

医疗卫生体系的主要目标有以下两类：

1. 临床目标，类似于传统临床活动的目标，如"准确快速地进行诊断"；

2. 人群目标，涉及整个人群的资源利用情况；临床医生在为一个体系制定指标时会经常忽视此群体指标。

专栏6.4列举了制定医疗卫生体系宏观目的的实操步骤，专栏6.5列举了就医疗卫生体系一系列具体目标达成一致所需要的实操步骤。在同一次会议上，负责体系开发的团队还应起草并就设立一系列目标达成共识。在设定目标的过程中，其范围可能需要调整。例如，在由公共卫生专业人员主持召开

changed. For example, when the draft set of objectives for liver disease were discussed in a workshop run by public health professionals, an objective to prevent liver disease, was introduced as follows:

To prevent alcoholic liver disease, principally by changing culture and the environment.

Box 6.4 Practical steps in the development of an aim for a system

- Hold a meeting of the management team
- Give the team the examples of aims shown in Box 6.3
- Ask people to work in pairs for 3 minutes to draft an aim for the system in development; then ask each pair for suggestions during feedback — it may be possible to reach agreement on a draft aim after one round of feedback but two or more rounds may be needed
- After feedback, draft an aim — redraft it if necessary and reach agreement; try to keep the length to under 25 words
- Circulate the draft aim to a wide range of stakeholders who will be involved in the system; give stakeholders and participants who attended the drafting meeting a month in which to respond
- Redraft the aim in the light of responses and suggested amendments

Box 6.5 Practical steps in the development of a set of objectives for a system

- Remind the group of the system aim that was previously agreed
- Consider circulating a draft set of objectives for another condition, for example, the objectives shown in Box 6.3 could be used, but from experience it is better to let people think freely
- Ask pople to work in pairs to identify at least one objective for the system in development
- Take feedback
- Type up the responses during a refreshment break
- At this stage, it may be necessary to introduce population-type objectives

Present the set of objectives and facilitate a discussion on each to reach an agreement on wording

■ Choosing criteria

For each objective, there should be one or more criteria associated with it to enable progress towards the objective to be measured. Choosing criteria is a more time-consuming process and may need to be addressed separately. For instance, it is important to reach an agreed definition of what is meant by certain phrases 'to diagnose quickly' and 'to diagnose accurately'.

的研讨会上，在针对预防肝病提出了目标：

主要通过改变文化和环境预防酒精性肝病。

专栏6.4 制定体系目的的实操步骤

- 召开管理团队会议。
- 给团队提供一个如专栏6.3所示的目的范例。
- 要求与会者分组工作3分钟，为拟开发的体系起草目的；然后在反馈过程中询问每一对工作小组的建议——有可能在讨论反馈后就可以对目的草案达成一致，但也可能需要两轮或者更多轮次的反馈。
- 在得到反馈后，起草一份目的——必要时重新起草并达成一致；尽量将字数控制在25个以内。
- 将草拟的目的分发给未来该体系的参与方，给他们和与会者一个月的时间进行回应。
- 根据收到的反馈和相关修改建议修订体系目的。

专栏6.5 制定体系目标的实操步骤

- 让与会人员了解之前已商定的体系目的。
- 可考虑向与会人员提供针对另一种情况制定一套目标草案作为参考，例如，可以使用专栏6.3中所示的目标，但根据既往经验，最好让人们自由思考。
- 安排与会者结对分组讨论，为正在开发中的体系确定至少一个具体目标。
- 回收反馈意见。
- 在茶歇期间整理录入反馈信息。
- 在此阶段，可能有必要引入人群层面的目标。

  整理出各组提出的目标后发给大家，逐一进行讨论并在措辞上达成一致。

■ 选择指标（Criteria）

对于每个具体目标，都应该有一个或多个与之相关的指标，目的是为了衡量该具体目标的进展情况。选择指标是一个非常耗时的过程，可能需要单独处理。例如，对"快速诊断"和"准确诊断"的定义达成一致是很重要的。

Each objective needs to have one or more criteria associated with it in order to measure progress. Without criteria, objectives are meaningless. Several terms are used as synonyms for 'criteria', such as 'metrics', 'indicators', or 'measures'. Some people use the term 'measures' to mean criteria that are considered to be of greater validity than indicators; for example, they would use the term 'measure' about systematic surveys of patient experience, whereas they would use the word 'indicator' for the number of letters of complaint or commendation that a hospital Chief Executive received. Although the latter is less costly, it is less valuable in terms of feedback for the system than the accurate measures used in the former.

Similar issues tend to be raised in any discussion about criteria that could be used to measure progress, including:

- *The availability of data*;
- *The validity of criteria*;
- *Whether to use process or outcome criteria.*

Availability of data

The data already being collected are rarely those needed to provide the information required to monitor progress, because originally they were selected for another specific reason. When selecting criteria, it is important not to be constrained by data availability, but to determine the criterion required to monitor each objective and then to specify the data needed to enable the measure to be calculated. For instance, if the criterion is related to the objective of diagnosing rheumatoid arthritis quickly, the data needed are:

- *the date of first presentation with joint pain*;
- *the date of definitive diagnosis.*

These data may be from different databases, the former in general practice records, of which there may be many of different types, the latter in hospital pharmacy records. In the past, this would have been a major problem because a new 'information system' would have had to be commissioned. Nowadays, and in future, however, the power of cloud computing, namely the ability to use the Internet as the storage system, enables data to be extracted from different sources.

每个具体目标都需要有一个或多个与之相关的指标以衡量进展。如果没有指标衡量，那具体目标就变得毫无意义。有几个术语常被用作"指标"的同义词，例如"矩阵（metrics）""指标（indicators）"或"度量标准（measures）"。有些人使用"度量标准"这个词来表示比指标更有效的标准；例如，他们会使用"度量标准"一词来表示对患者经历的系统性调查，而他们会使用"指数"一词来表示医院行政负责人收到的投诉或表扬信的数量。虽然后者的成本较低，但就对体系的反馈而言，它的价值不如前者所使用的测量方法准确。

在任何可用于衡量进展指标的讨论中，往往会提出类似的问题，包括：

● 数据的可获得性；

● 指标的有效性；

● 是使用过程指标还是结局指标。

数据的可获得性

已经收集到的数据往往不是监测进度所需的，因为最初收集这些数据是出于其他具体原因。在选择指标时，重要的是不要受数据可获得性的限制，而是要确定监测每个体系目标所需的指标，然后再确定用于计算指标所需的数据。例如，如果该指标与快速诊断类风湿性关节炎的目标相关，则需要的数据是：

● 首次出现关节疼痛的日期；

● 确诊日期。

这些数据可能来自不同的数据库，前者来自全科医生的诊疗记录，其中可能有许多不同类型，后者来自医院药房记录。这在过去可能是一个重要的问题，因为必须启用一个新的"信息系统"。然而现在乃至未来，我们可以借助云计算的力量，换言之，我们可以使用互联网作为存储系统，就可以从不同渠道提取数据。

Validity of criteria

The validity of a criterion is the degree to which it actually measures the change it purports to measure. For example, if one objective is to provide a service that patients value, the number of complaints received is of lower validity than a survey of all patients, although the latter is more time-consuming and more expensive to undertake.

This example demonstrates the trade-off between validity and feasibility: for a criterion with a high level of validity, the data are usually more difficult to collect than those for a criterion with a relatively low level of validity. If, however, the data for a criterion with a high level of validity become part of routine data collection, then services can be monitored using appropriate and what would usually be viewed as sophisticated measures. For instance, at the Dartmouth Hitchcock Medical Center, the preferences of each woman considering breast cancer treatment options are routinely collected which means that their recorded preference can then be compared with the treatment they actually receive.

■ Process or outcome criteria?

For decades, the provision of health services was measured using classic economic criteria such as the amount of resource invested or the volume of work done, i.e. inputs and outputs. In the 1960s, however, Avedis Donabedian published his work on quality assurance (5), and introduced a different nomenclature from that of the economists (see Table 6.3).

Table 6.3 A comparison of classic economic terminology and Donabedian's terminology in relation to healthcare criteria

Criterion	Economic terminology	Donabedian's terminology
Number of beds in surgical wards	Inputs	Structure
Number of operations in a year	Outputs	Process
Percentage of patients whose operation was a success	Not considered originally	Outcome
Use of resources	Outputs/inputs=productivity	Outcomes/inputs=efficiency

In the years following Donabedian's publication, there has been much discussion about the relative merits of process and outcome measures. Some authorities are proponents of outcome measures, whereas others support the use of process measures for the reason given by Porter.

指标的效度

一个指标的效度是指实际测量结果与真实情况之间的差异的程度。例如，如果一个具体目标是为患者提供满意的服务，则"收到的投诉数量"的效度要低于基于全部患者调查所获得的的指标，尽管后者更耗时且成本更高。

上述示例显示了指标效度和可行性之间的权衡：要获得效度高的指标，数据收集过程通常要难于准确性低的指标。但是，如果高效度指标的数据收集，能成为常规数据收集的一部分，则可将其用于监测服务，而且将作为优选指标使用。例如，达特茅斯希区柯克医疗中心会例行收集每位女性患者对乳腺癌治疗方案的偏好，这意味着可以将她们的偏好与其实际接受的治疗情况进行比较。

■ 过程指标还是结果指标？

几十年来，一直是使用经典的经济指标来衡量卫生健康服务的提供情况，例如投入的资源数量或完成的工作量，即投入和产出。然而在20世纪60年代，阿维迪斯·多纳贝迪安发表了他关于质量保证的著作[5]，并引入了与经济学家不同的命名法（表6.3）。

表6.3　医疗保健指标中的经典经济学术语和
多纳贝迪安术语的比较

指标	经济学术语	多纳贝迪安术语
外科病房的床位数量	投入	结构
一年内的手术数量	产出	过程
手术成功患者的百分比	最初不考虑	结局
资源使用情况	产出/投入＝生产率	结局/投入＝效率

在多纳贝迪安的著作发表之后的几年里，关于过程指标和结局指标的相对优点一直有很多讨论。一些权威机构支持结果指标，而另一些权威机构则基于波特给出的理由，支持使用过程指标。

There is a particular problem with outcomes in that it is often difficult to attribute a given outcome improvement (such as in the health of a patient) to a particular item of public service (such as a course of medical treatment), for the outcome may in large part be due to a variety of factors that are not within the control of the providers of the service concerned (such as the patient's own recuperative powers). This is one of the reasons why, although both providers and policy-makers often pay lip service to the important of outcomes, in practice they usually give more attention to factors that are more under the control of the service, such as inputs, processes and outputs.(6)

Currently, the trend is towards the measurement of outcomes, even if the criteria most readily available and easiest to collect are process measures.

Health outcomes refer to objective results, not just physician or patient perceptions of outcomes. There is not just one outcome of the care for any health condition, but multiple outcomes that jointly constitute value. Patient circumstances and preferences will affect the weighting of these outcomes to some degree....(7)

However, it is necessary to collect both outcome and process measures. Process measures remain important for two reasons:

1. the outcome of a service may not become apparent for years, rendering it unsuitable as a criterion for day-to-day management. The outcome of a breast cancer screening programme — such as a decline in mortality — will not become evident, even at a national level, for years, whereas the person responsible for managing a screening programme needs to know the outcome on an annual, monthly and sometimes, in the case of radiation levels, daily basis.

2. the outcome may be determined by factors other than the quality of the service. The practical steps that can be undertaken to select criteria for the monitoring of system objectives are shown in Box 6.6.

结局测量有一个特殊的问题，即通常很难将某一种结局的改善（例如患者的健康状况）归因于某一种特定的公共服务项目（例如医疗过程），因为这种结果可能在很大程度上归因于相关服务提供者无法控制的各种因素（例如患者自身的康复能力）。这就是为什么尽管服务的提供者和决策者经常口头应酬式地强调结果的重要性，但在实践中他们往往更关注服务中的可控因素，例如投入、过程和产出。[6]

目前的趋势是倾向于结局测量，即使过程测量是最容易获得和最容易收集的指标。

健康结局指的是客观的结果，而不仅是医生或患者对该结果的看法。对任何健康问题的照护都不止有一种结局，而是多种结局共同构成价值。患者自身状况及其个人偏好会在一定程度上影响这些结局的权重……[7]

然而，同时收集结局指标和过程指标的数据是非常有必要的。鉴于以下两个原因，过程指标仍然很重要：

1. 一项医疗服务的结局可能在数年内都无法明确体现，因此不适合作为日常管理的指标。如乳腺癌筛查计划的结局——死亡率的下降，即使在国家级层面上也可能很多年没有明显变化，而筛查项目的管理人员需要每年、每月甚至每天（如了解辐射水平），都要了解项目的进展。

2. 决定结局的因素可能并非医疗服务质量，而是其他多种因素。选择用于监测目标进展的指标的实际操作步骤见专栏6.6。

Box 6.6 Practical steps in the selection of criteria to monitor objectives in a system of care

- Invite the group involved in system development, involved in setting the objectives, and people with experience in designing research projects even if they are not doing research on the topic, their expertise in the definition and measurement of outcomes will be very helpful
- Prior to the meeting, conduct astructured literature search to identify outcome measures that are already available for the system focus
- If outcome measures are already available, in the meeting, consider whether to supplement them with outcomes of importance to your community of practice
- At the meeting, for each objective, ask participants to suggest the process criterion or criteria they would use to measure progress; reminding them not to take account at this stage of the availability or difficulty of obtaining the data necessary for monitoring
- Ask the professionals what constitutes a good outcome from their perspective and record the responses
- Ask the patients what constitutes a good outcome from their perspective and record the response
- Ask the professionals what constitutes a bad outcome from their perpective and record the responses
- Ask the patients what constitutes a bad outcome from their perspective and record the responses
- Ask the researchers to comment and advise on the responses of both professionals and patients
- Collate the responses about criteria, try to reach a consensus and record the conclusions
- Identify the data items associated with each criterion that are required to measure progress against the objectives, and specify the details relating to the data needed, the data collection cycle, and the adaptations to routine data systems that are necessary to enable data collection

■ Setting standards

A standard: the level of compliance with a criterion or indicator, for example 90% of patients in a practice with a blood pressure of more than 160/90 should have their blood pressure remeasured within three months.(8)

It is possible to set standards for a single system of care using the criteria and outcomes that have been agreed, including:

- *an excellent standard, the performance of the best service;*
- *a minimal acceptable standard, below which the system does not wish to fall;*
- *an achievable standard which can be arbitrarily, but usefully, set by choosing the cut-off point between the top quintile and the bottom three quintiles (Figure 6.4).*

专栏6.6　选择医疗服务体系目标监测指标的实际操作步骤

- 邀请参与体系开发和具体目标设定的团队，以及在设计研究项目方面有经验的人，即使他们没有进行过该领域的研究，但是他们在结局定义和测量方面的专业知识将会大有裨益。
- 在会议开始之前，进行结构化的文献检索，目的是找到已有的符合系统关注点的结局测量指标。
- 如果已有可用的结局测量指标，在会议上则需要考虑是否用社区实践的重要结果进行补充。
- 在会议中，请参会人员针对每一个具体目标提出测量进展过程的指标和他们愿意用的指标；同时要提醒他们无须考虑现阶段的数据可得性及获取难度。
- 询问专家从他们的角度来看什么是好的结局，并记录在册。
- 询问患者从他们的角度来看什么是好的结局，并记录在册。
- 询问专家从他们的角度来看什么是不良的结局，并记录在册。
- 询问患者从他们的角度来看什么是不良的结局，并记录在册。
- 请研究人员对专家和患者的反馈情况做出点评并提出建议。
- 收集关于指标的反馈意见，尽量达成共识并记录结果。
- 确定衡量目标进展所需的每个指标相关联的数据项目，并说明与所需数据相关的细节、数据收集周期，以及为实现数据收集所必需的对常规数据系统的调整。

■ 制定标准

标准：指某一指标的符合程度；例如90%血压超过160/90的患者应该在三个月内重新测量血压。[8]

可以使用已商定的指标和结果为单一医疗服务体系制定标准，包括：

- 卓越的标准，即最佳的服务表现；
- 最低可接受标准，即不希望体系失败的标准；
- 一个可实现的标准，可以任意设定，但通常是有助益地选择第一个五分位数（前20%）和最后三个五分位数（后60%）之间的界值作为衡量标准（图6.4）。

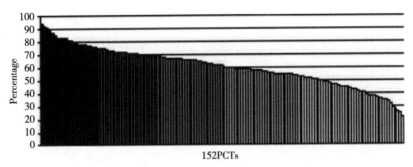

Figure 6.4 Percentage of patients admitted to hospital following a stroke who spend 90% of their time on a stroke unit by primary care trust (PCT) in England (2009/10) (9)

However, it is much better if several systems of care or services work together to set standards. One of the objectives of standard-setting is to help services improve their quality of care by competing with other services, using the standards as the benchmark. Standard-setting requires several services to apply the same objectives, criteria and standards — namely, to have a common system of care. If nationally agreed standards are available, these should be used; if there are no nationally agreed standards, follow the steps shown in Box 6.7. Once the system has been designed, the next stage is to build it. Building a system requires the development of a network of key organisations responsible for delivering care to the population.

Box 6.7 Practical steps towards standard-setting for a system of care

- Convene a meeting of the clinicians responsible for the population-based systems of care
- Prior to the meeting, identify the system objectives for which there are pre-existing good-quality performance information because, if possible, standards should be set using data that reflect the current situation across all the services; circulate this information prior to the meeting, but also ensure it is available at the meeting
- At the meeting, ask participants to consider the performance data for all the services, and to identify the performance level that constitutes a minimal acceptable standard for each objective
- Returning to the performance data, ask participants to identify the performance level that distinguishes the top quartile of sevices from the rest; agree this as the achievable standard towards which all services in the other three quartiles should aspire, the services in the top quartile to aspire to match, and the best performing service to try to do even better
- If there are no data that can be compared, ask participants to develop minimal acceptable and achievable standards based on their knowledge and experience

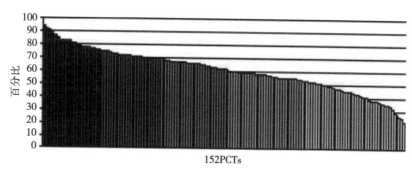

图6.4　在英国初级卫生保健信托机构中，脑卒中患者入院后90%住院时间在卒中病房的比例（2009年10月）[9]

　　然而，如果多个保健或服务体系共同制定标准则会达到更好的效果。制定标准的目标之一是在该标准的基础之上，通过与其他服务竞争，从而帮助服务部门提高服务质量。制定标准需要若干医疗卫生机构采用相同的目标、指标和标准——即具有一个共同的医疗卫生体系。如果有国家认可的标准，则应使用这些标准；如果没有国家认可的标准，请按照专栏6.7中所示的步骤制定标准。一旦体系设计完成，下一阶段就是如何构建。构建一个体系需要建立一个由为人群提供医疗服务的关键机构组成的网络。

专栏6.7　制定医疗卫生体系标准的实际操作步骤

- 召开临床医生会议，他们是为目标人群提供照护的责任主体。
- 会议开始前，尽量找出已有的拥有高质量绩效数据的体系目标，因为如有可能，应该用能够反映所有项目的当前所有情况的数据来制定标准；注意要在会议之前分享这些信息，并作为会议材料。
- 在会议中，请参会人员考虑所有服务的绩效数据，确定构成每个目标可接受的最低标准。
- 针对上述绩效数据，请参会人员将医疗服务水平划分成从高到低4个层次，将排名最靠前的服务水平设定为其余3个层次都应追求的可实现的标准；排名最靠前的医疗服务要尽力匹配到最佳水准，并追求更好的表现。
- 如果没有可比数据，请参会人员基于他们的经验和专业知识，设置可以接受并能实现的最低标准。

■ Questions for reflection or for use in teaching or network building

If using these questions in network building or teaching, put one of the questions to the group and ask them to work in pairs to reflect on the question for three minutes; try to get people who do not know one another to work together. When taking feedback, let each pair make only one point. In the interests of equity, start with the pair on the left-hand side of the room for responses to the first question, then go to the pair on the right-hand side of the room for responses to the second question.

- What are the main obstacles to the introduction and development of systems in healthcare?
- Identify five services including one that is diagnostic in which you are involved or which you know about, e.g. a service for women with pelvic pain. Give each of these services a score on a scale from 1 to 10, where 1 is chaos and 10 represents a perfect system.
- List three things that institutions are good at doing in healthcare and three things that they fail to do.

References

(1) Gray, J.A.M. (1983) Four Box Healthcare: Planning in a Time of Zero Growth. Lancet 2: 1185-1186.

(2) Grove, A.S. (1995) High output management. Vintage Books. (p.136)

(3) Scrivens, E. (2005) Quality, Risk and Control in Health Care. Open University Press (p.91).

(4) Drucker, P. (1955) The Practice of Management. Elsevier, Butterworth-Heinemann (p.54-55).

(5) Donabedian, A. (2003) Introduction to Quality Assurance in Healthcare. Oxford.

■ 互动思考题

如果在工作网络建设或教学中使用以下问题，可以将其中一个问题交给小组，让他们两人1组，思考3分钟，并尽量让彼此不认识的人一起工作。要求每组只能提出一个观点作为反馈。为了公平起见，让房间左侧的一组开始回答第1个问题，然后让房间右侧的一组开始回答第2个问题。

- 在引进和发展医疗卫生体系的过程中主要有哪些障碍？

- 确定5项医疗卫生服务，其中包括一项你本人所涉及或了解的诊断服务，如针对女性盆腔疼痛的医疗服务。给每项服务打分，评分范围从1到10，"1"代表混乱无序，"10"则代表该医疗服务体系完美无缺。

- 列出各医疗卫生机构在医疗服务领域中3件做得好的服务和3件未能做好的服务。

参 考 文 献

(6) Porter, M.E. (2008) What is Value in Health Care? Harvard Business School. Institute for Strategy and competitiveness. White Paper.

(7) Neumann, P.J., Tunis, S.R. (2010) Medicare and Medical Technology — the Growing Demand for Relevant Outcomes. New Eng. J. Med. 362: 5: 377.

(8) Grol, M., Baker, R., Moss, F. (2004) Quality Improvement Research. BMJ Books.

(9) Right Care (2010) NHS Atlas of Variation in Healthcare. Reducing unwarranted variation to increase value and improve quality. November 2010 (p.48). http://www.rightcare.nhs.uk/atlas

Chapter 7
CREATING NETWORKS TO DELIVER SYSTEMS

第七章
为供给体系建立工作网络

This chapter will:

- define networks and networking;
- describe the principles of network management;
- summarise steps that can be taken to build sustainable networks;
- give examples of different types of networks, classified by the degree of managerial formality;
- describe interventions that can be used to develop or strengthen the network;
- describe the need for explicit pathways that patients can follow through the network.

By the end of this chapter, you will have developed an understanding of:

- the difference between a network and a hierarchy;
- the relative contributions of institutions and systems;
- how to build a network;
- how to sustain and develop a network;
- the contribution that networks make to delivering systems of care;
- the role of a network coordinator;
- the difference between a network and a team;
- the contribution that pathways make to standardise and personalise care.

Once a system of care has been designed, the next step is to deliver it to the population in need. There are two principal ways in which change is brought about within a health service — through people or through the organisation, each of which comprises three elements (see Figure 7.1).

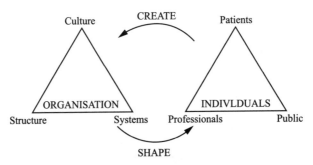

Figure 7.1 The two elements of a health service — the people and the organisation

本章涉及内容：

● 定义和建立工作网络；

● 介绍工作网络的管理原则；

● 总结建立可持续工作网络的步骤；

● 依据管理形式的等级进行分类，给出不同工作网络类型的例子；

● 说明可用于发展或加强工作网络的措施；

● 说明患者依照工作网络行事所需的明确路径。

在本章末，读者将会深入理解：

● 工作网络和等级制度之间的区别；

● 机构和体系各自所做出的贡献；

● 如何建立工作网络；

● 如何维持和发展工作网络；

● 工作网络对医疗卫生服务系统的贡献；

● 工作网络协调员的作用；

● 工作网络和团队之间的区别；

● 工作路径对标准化和个性化医疗卫生服务的贡献。

一旦医疗卫生服务体系设计完成，下一步就是将其应用于需要的人群。有两种主要方式可以使卫生服务体系发生变化——通过人群和组织，每种方式包括3个要素（图7.1）。

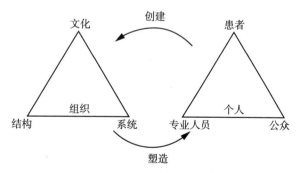

图7.1 卫生服务的两个要素——人群与组织

For the last 50 years, those who pay for or manage health services have sought to achieve change principally by changing the structure of the organisation, given that it can take years or decades for education to have an effect.

■ The need to shift the focus from structure

Organizing is the process of arranging collective effort so that it achieves an outcome potentially superior to that of individuals acting or working alone. It almost always involves some division of labor, with different people or groups concentrating on different activities that have to be integrated (co-ordinated) to achieve a successful result. (1)

In seeking to change the organisation of healthcare, priority has previously been given to changing the structure:

- *by re-organising the bureaucracy;*
- *by introducing a market;*
- *by both re-organisation and the introduction of a market.*

In this book, it is argued that priority should be given to the development of population-based and integrated systems of care rather than to structural change. Indeed, there is a growing consensus that a new form of organisation is needed to deliver a system of care.

This new form is known as a network, and will become the dominant type of organisation in the 21st century, displacing, but not rendering redundant, the bureaucracy, the dominant type of organisation in the 20th century.

As health services grew in size during the 20th century, it became clear that clinicians needed an organisation to support them. The type of organisation that flourished in every country's health service was the bureaucracy, much criticised by those who have experienced only bad bureaucracy. Bureaucratisation, however, can bring several benefits.

'Bureaucracy' is a dirty word, both to the average person and to many specialists on organizations. It suggests rigid rules and regulations, a hierarchy of offices, narrow specialization of personnel, an abundance of offices or units which can hamstring those who want to get things done, impersonality, resistance to change. Yet every organization of any significant size is bureaucratized to some degree or, to put it differently, exhibits more or less stable patterns of behaviour based upon a structure of roles and specialized tasks. Bureaucracy, in this sense, is another word for structure. (2)

基于教育可能需要几年或几十年才能产生效果，在过去50年中，卫生服务的支付方或管理者主要是通过改变组织结构来进行改革。

■ 将注意力从结构转移的需求

组织工作是一个集合多方力量的过程，这样才会取得可能优于个体行为或独自工作的结果。它一般涉及不同的人或团体的分工，分别专注于不同的活动，需要将其有机整合或协调才能取得最后的成功。[1]

在医疗卫生服务的组织机构寻求变革时，以往优先通过以下几个方面对结构进行改变：

- 重组政府管理体系；
- 引入市场机制；
- 以上两种方式并用。

本书论证了相对于改变医疗卫生体系的结构，应该优先发展基于人群的整合型医疗服务体系。事实上，医疗卫生体系需要建立新的组织形式，这一点已得到业内越来越多的共识。

这种新形式即工作网络。工作网络将成为21世纪医疗卫生体系的主要形式，取代20世纪以政府体系为主的管理体制，且不会再增加一些冗余工作。

20世纪期间，随着医疗服务规模的扩大，临床医生需要一个组织来提供支持其需求的事实越来越明显了。在所有国家的医疗服务中占据主导地位的组织类型是政府体系，那些仅对政府为主导的体制有过不良体验的人对其进行了很多批评。然而，政府体系也可以带来几点益处。

对普通人和许多组织中的专家而言，"官僚主义"是一个贬义词。它意味着僵化的规章制度、办公室的等级制度、个人专业知识的局限性、大量的办公室或部门，这会降低那些想把事情做好的人的工作效率、无人情味以及抵触改变等。然而，任何大型规模的组织多多少少都存在官僚主义，换言之，在职能结构和业务工作的基础上，表现出或多或少固化的行为模式。从这个意义上说，官僚主义是（组织）结构的代名词。[2]

Although bureaucracies are necessary, they can develop in ways that are unhelpful if they have misguided leadership. One manifestation of over-bureaucratisation is an emphasis on hierarchy, i.e. 'a system of nested groups' (3), in which senior managers operate in what is known as 'command and control' mode.

Markets have also been introduced to varying degrees in the organisation of health services in many countries: in the United States, the role of the market is extensive, whereas in Canada that role is much less. Thus, in the last 50 years, both bureaucracies and markets have come to dominate the delivery of healthcare.

■ The network, a new type of organisation for healthcare

A new type of organisation for the delivery of healthcare is evolving, known as a network:

Networking is a broad concept referring to a form of organized transacting that offers an alternative to either markets or hierarchies. It refers to transactions across an organization's boundaries that are recurrent and involve continuing relationships with a set of partners. The transactions are coordinated and controlled on a mutually agreed basis that is likely to require common protocols and systems, but do not necessarily require direct supervision by the organization's own staff. (1)

Debate often arises about whether the word 'network' is a noun or a verb. The definition of 'networking' in the quotation above summarises the fact that a network is both an entity and an activity, as well as being a gerund, a 'doing' word.

Networks as organisations are different from hierarchies. As emphasized by Wright, networks are not 'top down'.

A network...emerges from the bottom up; individuals function as autonomous nodes, negotiating their own relationships, forging ties, coalescing into clusters. There is no 'top' in a network; each node is equal and self-directed. Democracy is a kind of network; so is a flock of birds, or the World Wide Web. (3)

Wright's definition of a network introduces the term 'node', which also helps to differentiate networks from hub-and-spoke organisations. A hub-and-spoke organisation implies that one partner is more important than the others, whereas in

虽然有时官僚体系是必要的，但是如果领导力受其负面影响，则对其自身发展是无益的。过度官僚化的一个表现就是强调等级制度，例如：在某种群体中，上级管理者只会使用"指挥－控制"的方式来推进工作。

在许多国家，市场机制都不同程度地被引入了卫生服务体系。在美国，市场的作用十分广泛；而在加拿大，市场的作用则小得多。在过去50年中，官僚体制和市场机制均主导了医疗卫生服务体系的运行。

■ 工作网络——一种医疗卫生体系的新型组织形式

一种新型的医疗卫生的组织形式正在发展壮大，即工作网络：

> 工作网络从广义上讲，是指一种有组织的业务来往方式，为市场机制或等级制度提供了替代方案。工作网络是超越某个机构（专业、职能）范围之外与其他一些合作伙伴的经常、持续的交往。这种业务往来基于合作伙伴之间的共识来共同协作管理，有可能需要遵循统一的操作规范和工作流程，但不一定需要组织内部成员直接监督管理。[1]

关于"工作网络"是一个名词还是一个动词的问题经常引起一些争论。上述引文中"工作网络"的定义概括了一个事实，即工作网络既是一个实体、一项活动，也是一个动名词，即一个"活动正在进行中"的动名词。

工作网络的组织形式和等级管理制度是不同的，如怀特所说，工作网络不是"自上而下"的管理方式。

> 工作网络是自下而上产生的，个体充当自治节点，协商彼此关系，建立合作纽带并集结成群落。在工作网络中没有上级领导，每一个节点都是平等的、自主的。所谓"民主"就是一种"网络"，一群鸟或万维网都是某种形式的工作网络。[3]

怀特在工作网络的定义中引入了"节点"一词，以此区分工作网络和中心辐射式组织。中心辐射式组织意味着其中一个合作伙伴比其他都重要，而

a network all the partners — the professor, the generalist, and the patient — are all 'nodes' of equal importance but have different roles.

■ Networks and teams

Within a bureaucracy, teams play a very important part in delivering care. The importance of good teamwork, particularly multidisciplinary teamwork, is increasingly being recognised. A new term was developed by Paul Batalden and colleagues at Dartmouth Hitchcock Medical Center — the clinical microsystem — defined as:

...the sharp end of care — the places where care is actually delivered in the real world. We call these small frontline systems of care clinical microsystems. They are literally the places where patients and families and care teams meet. (4)

There are, however, important differences between teams, including multidisciplinary teams, and clinical microsystems and networks. Networks differ from teams in at least three ways (see Display 7.1).

Display 7.1

Teams	*Networks*
● Members all work in the same organisation	● Members come from different organisations
● Communication is primarily face-to-face	● Face-to-face contact is usually infrequent
● One member is usually designated as the person who has bureaucratic authority by the organisation in which the team works	● It is uncommon for one person to have bureaucratic control

Networks are developed through sapiential authority, that is, an authority based on knowledge, originally defined by Max Weber more than a century ago. Although the leadership of a team can also be strengthened by sapiential or charismatic authority, the designation of one clinician as the clinical director of a department does not necessarily confer all the authority that the person may need. The person designated may not be the most experienced clinician; indeed, they may be the only one willing to do the job. If, however, that person was appointed because they have the right personality for the job, they will be able to generate the necessary charisma.

工作网络中所有的合作伙伴——包括教授、全科医生和患者这些"节点"——都同样重要，但是发挥不同的作用。

■ 工作网络和团队

在官僚体系中，团队在提供医疗卫生服务方面有着十分重要的作用。团队合作的重要性，特别是多学科团队合作，越来越得到业界的认可。达特茅斯大学希区柯克医学中心的 Paul Batalden 及其同事发明了一个新术语，"临床微系统"，定义为：

> ……医疗卫生服务的前端——现实中医疗卫生服务供给的场所。我们称这些小型前端卫生服务供给系统为临床微系统，实际上就是患者、家庭和卫生服务团队会面的场所。[4]

然而，多学科团队、临床微系统和工作网络之间都存在着重要的差异。工作网络与团队至少在3个方面有所不同（场景7.1）。

场景7.1　团队和工作网络的区别

团队	工作网络
所有成员都在一个机构工作	成员均来自不同的机构
主要通过面对面交流	面对面交流通常不是很频繁
一个成员被机构指定为负责人来领导团队的工作	一般不会指定一个负责人

在一个多世纪前，马克斯·韦伯最初定义工作网络是通过智慧权威（即基于知识的权威性）发展而来的。尽管团队领导力也可以通过智慧权威或者魅力权威得以加强，但任命一位临床医生为科室主任并不意味着赋予其全部权威。被任命的人员可能不是最有经验的临床医生；事实上，他们可能是愿意做这项工作的唯一人选。而如果此类人员确实是由于胜任而被任命的，则他们可以展现必要的魅力。

■ Types of network

Although networks run primarily on trust rather than hierarchical authority, some of the relationships within a network are governed by formal rules of conduct, or sometimes contracts. The Royal College of Paediatrics and Child Health (RCPCH) defined four types of network depending on the degree of formality (see Box 7.1).

Box 7.1 Four types of network identified by the RCPCH (5)

Clinical Association: an informal group that corresponds or meets to consider clinical topics, best practice and other areas of interest

Clinical Forum: a more formal group than a clinical association that meets regularly and has an agenda that focuses on clinical topics; there is an agreement to share audit and formulate jointly agreed clinical protocols

Developmental Network: a clinical forum that has started to develop a broader focus other than purely clinical topics, with an emphasis on service improvement

Managed Clinical Network: includes the function of a clinical forum, but has a formal management structure with defined governance arrangements and specific objectives linked to a published strategy

The evolution of Accountable Care Organisations

In several countries, a more formal split has been established between organisations that pay for healthcare, such as insurance companies, and those who provide healthcare. In NHS England, it is the role of commissioner to pay for healthcare. With the development of this formal split, a type of network is emerging that has a greater degree of bureaucratic, contractual formality than has been the case hitherto. The term for such an organisation in the United States is the Accountable Care Organisation (ACO).

ACOs consist of providers who are jointly held accountable for achieving measured quality improvements and reductions in the rate of spending growth. Our definition emphasizes that these cost and quality improvements must achieve overall, per capita improvements in quality and cost, and that ACOs should have at least limited accountability for achieving these improvements while caring for a defined population of patients. (6)

■ 工作网络的类型

尽管工作网络的运作主要靠彼此的信任而非等级关系，网络内机构之间的关系通常也需要受到正式的行为准则或合同制约。皇家儿科和儿童健康学院（RCPCH）根据正式程度定义了4种网络类型（专栏7.1）。

专栏7.1 RCPCH定义的4种工作网络类型[5]

- 临床协会：非正式小组，通过通信方式或会议来讨论临床主题、最佳实践和其他感兴趣领域。
- 临床论坛：是比临床协会更为正式的小组，定期召开会议，制定聚焦于临床主题的议程；双方就共享审计达成一致意见，并共同制定一致的临床行事规则。
- 发展型的工作网络：临床论坛，开始扩展到更广泛的关注点，而不再是纯临床的主题，其重点是改善服务。
- 管理临床管理工作网络：包括临床论坛的功能，但具有正式的管理结构、有明确的管理规定和与公布的战略相关的具体目标。

责任医疗组织的演变

在一些国家，医疗卫生服务的支付机构（如保险公司）和服务机构已经正式分开。在NHS中，特定的行政长官负责支付医疗卫生的相关费用。在医疗卫生服务的支付机构和服务机构正式分离的过程中，形成了一种更加繁复、更拘泥于合同形式的工作网络。在美国，这类机构叫作"责任医疗组织"（ACO）。

ACO是由一批医疗供给者组成，他们共同负责实现医疗质量收益和卫生支出增长率的降低。我们的定义强调，必须有能力统筹实现成本和质量的改进，即人均成本和质量的改进。责任医疗组织为特定患者群体提供服务的同时，应该为提高质量和降低成本负有有限的责任。[6]

The term Accountable Care Organisation has been used in the NHS although it has not been generally adopted. There is agreement, however, about the need to develop networks that have more formality than groups of professionals who have a common interest.

One model is for one service to be given a contract to act as the 'prime contractor' or 'prime provider', responsible for involving all the other relevant services and, where necessary, issuing a subcontract. This type of organisation:

- *is responsible for ensuring that integrated care is delivered to a defined population within a fixed budget to explicit quality standards and outcomes*;
- *will need a lead clinician skilled in population medicine, one of whose responsibilities will be to produce an explicit care pathway or care map which most patients should follow through the network.*

Another approach is for payers to change the type of contract they use. Traditionally, payers contracted with the main islands in the archipelago of healthcare — hospitals, primary care, community services and mental health services (see Figure 6.1). Such contracts have focused on price and volume supported by a few quality indicators, such as waiting list times. A new approach uses population-and outcomes-based incentivised contracts so that all the relevant clinicians from the different provider organisations are incentivised to work together focused on the needs of, for example, all the people with musculoskeletal disease in a population.

Practical steps in building an effective network for integrated care

When developing a network for integrated care, several variables can influence what it is possible to achieve, including:

- *the management style of the health service, for example, has it adopted the principle of the Accountable Care Organisation with a lead contractor*;
- *the degree to which the network is related to a system of care with a clear, written plan recognised by the principal organisations involved*;

ACO这个名词曾经在NHS使用过，不过没有被广泛采纳。然而，业界一致认为有必要建立一种更加正式的工作网络，而非仅靠一些兴趣相投的专业团队在一起工作。

这种ACO的一种运作模式是把其中一个机构作为"主合同方"或"主要供给方"与其签订合同，负责统筹其他参与机构的工作，并在必要时与其他机构签订子合同。这类机构：

- 负责确保在固定的预算范围内，按照明确的质量标准和结果，向特定的人群得到整合型医疗服务；
- 需要由精通群医学的临床医生领导，其职责之一是建立清楚明确的医疗卫生服务路径或路线图，让大部分患者可通过工作网络接受医疗服务。

另外一种方式是由支付方来改变他们的合约类型。传统方式是支付方和众多医疗卫生保健供给方中的主体部分（如医院、初级卫生保健机构、社区服务机构及精神卫生机构，图6.1）等签订合同，这类合同侧重于价格及数量，并铺之以一些质量指标，如预约等候时间。新的运作方式是签订基于人群和服务结果的、具有激励机制的合同，激励所有相关的来自不同医疗卫生提供方的临床医生共同努力，来满足人群中的特定疾病患者的服务需求，如肌肉骨骼系统疾病患者。

建立有效运行工的整合型医疗保健工作网络的实践步骤

在建立整合型医疗卫生服务网络时，以下几个因素会影响其工作效果：

- 医疗卫生服务的管理模式，例如，它是否采用了包含主要承包商的ACO原则；
- 工作网络与医疗卫生体系关联整合的程度。此体系拥有被主要参与机构所认可的清晰的书面计划；

- *the degree of authority given to the person charged with leading or coordinating the network;*
- *the support provided to the individual identified as the coordinator, for example, has the coordinator been given protected time and secretarial support to arrange meetings, or information scientist support to create a website and a virtual community?*

These are the issues that the participating organisations need to discuss. The outcomes of such discussions are likely to be determined by the level of trust the organisations have in one another. There are, however, some general steps that can be taken when building a network to deliver integrated care (see Box 7.2).

Box 7.2 Practical steps in building a network for integrated care, assuming the objectives, criteria and standards have been agreed

- Identify the key constituencies
- Within each constituency, identify the person with power and the person most likely to participate enthusiastically in the network – they may not be the same person
- Involve both patient and carer organisations
- Seek resources for a first meeting of the network; consider asking an influential speaker to the launch
- Ask people to introduce themselves
- Ask participants to work in pairs with someone whom they have not met before to discuss the systems document for five minutes and address the question "What are the priorities that the network should tackle in our first year?"
- Ask people to work in pairs, but this time with a different person whom they have not met before, to address the question 'How could the network be enjoyable and productive?' (For example, how often should we have face-to-face meetings, should we have webinars, is there a place for speakers, either from within the participating organisations or from outside?)

Maintaining the network for integrated care

Networks are dynamic and once set up they need nurturing. The person appointed as network coordinator has the responsibility for maintaining the network. Practical steps to help maintain a network for integrated care are shown in Box 7.3.

● 工作网络领导者或协调者的权限大小；

● 协调者得到的支持程度，例如，是否保障协调者有足够的时间及足够的行政和信息技术支持来组织会议，或是否有信息技术专家的支持以建立网站和虚拟社区？

以上这些因素，需要参与机构仔细讨论。而讨论的结果可能取决于组织之间的信任程度。然而，在建立工作网络以提供整合型医疗服务时，需要实施几个基本步骤（专栏7.2）。

专栏7.2　在明确目标、准则和标准前提下，建立整合型
医疗工作网络的实践步骤

● 确定主要区域。

● 在每个区域内，确定有决策权力的人和最有可能积极参与到工作网络的人——他们可能不是同一个人。

● 由患者和医疗卫生服务机构共同参与。

● 为第一次工作网络会议寻找资源：考虑邀请一位有影响力的演讲者出席启动会。

● 请每个人做自我介绍。

● 使参与者与其从未结识过的人两两结伴，花5分钟讨论，讨论"工作网络在第一年应该优先解决的事项是什么？"。

● 但是这一次，让人们与另一个他不认识的人两两结伴，但是这一次换另一个人，并讨论"工作网络如何变得令人愉悦和富有成效？"（例如，我们应该多久举行一次面对面的会议，是否应该举办网络研讨会，来自组织内部或外部的演讲者是否有发言的机会？）。

维护整合型医疗工作网络

工作网络是动态的，一旦建立就需要维护。任命为工作网络协调员的人有责任去维护工作网络。有助于维护整合型医疗工作网络的实践步骤见专栏7.3。

Box 7.3 Steps to help maintain the network

- Aim to make all meetings educational, and ensure participants are able to claim points for continuing professional development for either all or part of the meeting
- Buddy up with another network, pethaps not one which is a contiguous competitor, and encourage exchange visits by either the whole network or individuals
- Use the Annual Report as an opportunity for reflection, goalsetting, and motivation
- Encourage the conduct of research projects that involve the network as a whole
- Deal with hostile or unenthusiastic members directly and quickly; enlisting the help of their line manager may be helpful.Always bear in mind the adage: 'When deciding whether to be paranoid or puzzled, choose puzzled — it is much more effective'

■ Ending the era of primary and secondary care

For the specialist who has responsibility for a population and is developing a network, it is vital to create a culture in which everyone is considered to be of equal importance. This is not always easy to achieve:

- *medicine has become split into primary and secondary care, which can be counterproductive when building a system;*
- *even in the United Kingdom where primary care or general practice is acknowledged as having the same intellectual standing as any secondary care or hospital specialty, a prejudice remains that general practitioners are of lower status.*

This prejudice is reinforced when the issue of 'missed diagnosis' in general practice is raised by hospital specialists or of over-use of resources raised by general practitioners.

'It was an easy diagnosis. How did those guys miss it?'
—Hospital doctor speaking about general practitioners
'Why do they keep doing all these tests? They've lost their clinical judgment?'
—General practitioners speaking about hospital doctors

Although such criticism is sometimes justified, it is usually made by a clinician who is not familiar with the difference between sensitivity and positive predictive value (see Box 7.4). Moreover, this criticism highlights an important con-

专栏7.3　有助于维护工作网络的步骤

- 旨在使所有会议都能起到教育作用，让参会者能够在会议整个进程或部分环节中，随意发表观点，得到持续专业发展。
- 与另一个或许没有竞争关系的工作网络建立伙伴关系，并鼓励整个工作网络或个人进行交流访问。
- 可将年度报告作为深入思考、设定目标和激励的机会。
- 鼓励开展涉及整个工作网络的研究项目。
- 当遇到那些对工作抵触或没有热情的成员，如何面对或快速解决存在的问题时，获取他们部门负责人的支持可能会有帮助。要记住这样的格言："在过分猜疑和装糊涂之间，往往选择装糊涂效果更好"。

■ 初级和二级卫生保健割裂的时代结束

对人群健康负有责任、要建立医疗卫生保健网络的专科医生来说，创立一种每个人都同等重要的文化氛围十分重要。这不是很容易做到，因为：

- 医学已经被分割成初级卫生保健和二级卫生保健，这两部分在建立卫生服务体系时可能是互相抵触的；
- 即使在英国，初级医疗或全科医生被认为与任何二级医疗或医院专科具有相同的知识地位，但全科医生地位较低的偏见依然存在。

当专科医生指出全科医疗中出现"漏诊"问题，或者全科医生认为专科医生过度使用资源时，这种偏见更被强化了。

- "这种疾病很容易诊断，那些医生怎么能漏诊呢？"

　　　　　　　　　　　　　　　　　——医院的专科医生谈论全科医生时说

- "为什么他们总是做这么多化验检查呢？他们连最基本的临床判断都没有吗？"　　　　　　　　——全科医生又会说医院的专科医生

尽管类似指责有时也不无道理，但这种指责通常出自不懂灵敏度和阳性预测值区别的临床医生之口（专栏7.4）。此外，这种指责凸显了群医学中的

sideration in population medicine regarding the different perspectives of clinicians who are providing different types of care for people in the population served:

- *the perspective of the clinician in primary care or general practice, who is the first point of contact for the general population*;
- *the perspective of the clinician in secondary care, who sees only those patients who have been filtered for referral by the clinician who was the first point of contact — these patients represent a subset of the population.*

As the prevalence of disease in the general population is different from that in the population subset who have been referred, the positive predictive value for every test is different.

Box 7.4 Definitions of sensitivity and positive predictive value

- *Sensitivity*: the proportion of people with the disease who are identified as having it by a positive test result
- *Positive predictive value*: the probability that a person with a positive test result actually has the disease (7)

Furthermore, the neurosurgeon who says that haemorrhagic stroke is an 'easy' diagnosis because all the patients reaching the service complain of atypical headache in middle age is failing to appreciate that, although almost all of the patients who have had a stroke will report that they had an atypical headache, if every general practitioner referred every patient with atypical headache the specialist service would collapse.

In building a community of practice, it may be more helpful to talk of generalists and specialists, but this terminology could also have pejorative connotations. Although specialists may know more about a particular specialty, it is important to recognise that specialists and generalists are dealing with different subgroups within the whole population served.

When building a system of care and creating a community of practice to work within that system, it is important to encourage a culture change in which people refer to all the clinicians serving a population, and the terms primary and secondary care are made redundant.

一个重点考虑因素，即为患者人群提供不同类型医疗卫生服务的临床医生们的不同视角：

- 初级卫生保健或全科医生的临床医生视角：这些医生通常是一般大众最先接触的医务工作者；
- 二级卫生保健医生的视角：他们仅诊治那些经过初级卫生保健医生初步"筛选"或转诊的患者，这些患者代表了人群的一部分。

疾病的患病率在普通人群和被转诊的那部分人群中是不同的，因此每种检测的阳性预测值是不同的。

专栏7.4　灵敏度和阳性预测值的定义

- 灵敏度：实际患病且其试验结果为阳性的百分比。
- 阳性预测值：一个检查结果为阳性的人其实际患该病的可能性。[7]

此外，神经外科医生认为出血型脑卒中"很容易诊断"，是因为在专科被诊断为脑卒中的中年患者都出现非典型性头痛；这些神经外科医生没有意识到，虽然确诊为脑卒中的所有患者几乎都报告有非典型性头痛，但如果全科医生把每一位有非典型性头痛的患者都转诊给他们，专科医疗服务就会崩溃。

在构建医疗卫生服务共同体时，用全科医生和专科医生这样的名词可能会更有帮助，尽管这两个术语的使用有时略带贬义。专科医生可能在某一特定领域了解得更多，但重要的是要意识到，专科医生和全科医生是为总人群中的不同群体服务的。

在构建医疗卫生保健体系和建立医疗卫生保健共同体时，重要的是鼓励转变人们认为所有医生均照护同一人群并且初级卫生和二级卫生这类术语实则多余的文化误区。初级卫生保健和二级卫生保健这类术语实则多余。

■ Making care pathways

As the delivery of care becomes more complicated, both patients and clinicians can benefit from care pathways, which describe the path a patient with a particular problem usually follows through the network. The term 'care pathways' or 'integrated care pathways' (ICP), however, is used in different ways. A team in Scotland has identified three different meanings associated with the term integrated care pathway (see Box 7.5), and although they believe all three meanings are valid considerations when developing pathways they would argue that only point 3 represents an integrated care pathway and suggest that points 1 and 2 are called 'pathways of care'.(8)

Box 7.5　Different meanings attributed to the term 'integrated care pathway' (8)

1. The actual care process experienced by each individual patient/client; in the literature, this is represented as a journey in which the patient/client is the traveller

2. Maps that define best practice and the minimum clinical standards or essential components of care for every patient/client in a given situation: a care pathway is a standard or universal plan for how a patient/client with a particular condition will be treated

3. Physical documentation located at the point of care which may replace traditional records, also called the care pathway: central to the task of patient/client care under the pathway approach, as the care process is clearly presented on the documentation for all those involved to see

Depicting the care pathway using software such as the Map of Medicine helps develop a common understanding of the aims and objectives of the system and contributes to the collective memory of the system. The system of care can be regarded as a neural network, which is based on knowledge.

■ Resistance to the development of care pathways

There has been professional resistance to the development of care pathways which some clinicians claim will lead to standardisation or 'cookbook' medicine. Although such criticisms need to be addressed, one powerful way to tackle widespread unwarranted variation in clinical practice is through the use of care pathways. In addition, standardisation of certain aspects of clinical care enables the inexperienced clinician to concentrate on an individual patient's anxieties and concerns and to personalise the patient's care, rather than trying to remember which post-operative fluid regime a particular surgeon prefers. Standardisa-

■建立照护路径

由于提供医疗卫生服务的模式越来越复杂，患者和医生都可以从照护路径上获益。照护路径即一个有特定疾病的患者在医疗卫生的工作网络内通常要遵循的路径。然而，"照护路径"和"整合型照护路径（ICP）"两个名词的使用方法不同。一个苏格兰团队提出了"整合型照护路径"这一术语的3个不同含义（专栏7.5）。尽管在建立路径时他们认为这3个含义都是合理的，但他们声称只有第3点才代表了"整合型照护路径"，而建议把第1点和第2点称为"照护路径"。[8]

专栏7.5　整合型照护路径的不同含义 [8]

1. 每个患者实际所经历的照护过程：用文学语言可以描述为一次旅行，而每个患者就是一个旅行者。
2. 路径图就是每个患者在特定情况下可得到的最佳照护以及该照护的最低临床标准或必要组成内容：单个照护路径是有特定疾病患者所接受治疗的规范化或通用型方案。
3. 患者接受照护过程中，在每个照护节点都有记录首要任务的实物文档。过程、路径中的各个节点以及预期的进展都会清晰地记录在文档中，以供所有相关人员参考。

用医学路径图这样的软件描绘照护路径有助于对建立该系统的目的和目标形成共识，并有助于系统的集体记忆。医疗卫生服务体系可以看作是一个基于知识的神经网络。

■建立照护路径的阻碍

在建立照护路径时，存在一些来自专业人员的阻力，一些临床医生认为这会导致标准化医疗或"按图索骥式"医疗。尽管批评者提出的问题要予以解决，但要解决临床工作中普遍存在的不合理差异化的问题，一种有效的方法就是使用照护路径。此外，临床照护中某些方面采取标准化操作可使那些经验不足的临床医生能更专注于处理患者个体焦虑和担忧的情绪，为患者提供个性化的服务，而不必费心记住一些无关紧要之事，如某个外科医生更喜

tion is particularly important therefore when care is delivered by inexperienced clinicians.

Another reason why standardisation of clinical care has been resisted is because some clinicians see it as a political process.

...standardization is a thoroughly political enterprise in at least two ways. First of all, standardization is political in the sense that the process of standardization is typified by ongoing negotiations between a host of actors, none of whom is in control or oversees all issues that may be at stake....Second, standardization is political since it inevitably reorders practices, and such reorderings have consequences that affect the position of actors (through, for example, the distribution of resources and responsibilities). (9)

Although this view of standardisation can be justified because the implementation of standardisation will affect clinical freedom, to oppose standardisation when there is incontrovertible evidence of unwarranted variation in clinical practice is politically naïve.

Clinicians who defend clinical freedom fail to appreciate that there are two types of freedom, distinguished by Isaiah Berlin in his essay Two Concepts of Liberty (10):

- *negative liberty, the freedom for every individual clinician to decide on every process of care;*
- *positive liberty, the amount of freedom a profession has to decide how much negative liberty its members should have.*

Many people who fight for negative liberty fail to see that it is more advantageous to maintain 'positive liberty'. Professional organisations need to be at the forefront of standardising clinical practice, or else, in defence of negative liberty, they will sacrifice positive liberty, that freedom which it is most important to possess.

The way in which pathways are introduced can reduce the level of resistance. For example, when localising a pathway, expressed using the Map of Medicine, it is important to emphasise that it needs to be adapted for the local population. Some items in the pathway need to be localised, such as the names and contact details of key local services. Some items should not be varied, such as the prescription of a drug which is supported by very strong evidence and national guidance. However, there are often steps in the pathway that can be changed because of some local circumstance, such as the opportunity to offer a patient entry into a randomised controlled trial.

欢用那种术后输液方案。标准化对于经验不足的临床医生提供医疗卫生照护时尤为重要。

临床照护标准化面临阻力的另一个原因是，一些临床医生认为它被政治化了。

> ……至少从两个方面可以看出临床照护标准化是一个彻头彻尾的政治过程。首先，标准化的典型特征是，许多参与者之间进行谈判，但没有一个参与者对所有可能关乎风险的问题起控制或监督作用……从这个意义上来说标准化即是政治化了。其次，标准化是政治化了的原因，是因为它不可避免地要重新规划实践流程，而这种重新排序的结果会导致参与者的地位发生变化（例如，通过资源和责任的再分配）。[9]

尽管认为标准化的实施会影响临床自由度的观点是合理的，但当临床实践中存在不合理问题证据确凿时，反对标准化是政治上不够成熟的表现。

主张临床自主权的临床医生没有意识到，自由分为两种类型，这在伊赛亚·伯林的《两种自由概念》的文章[10]中做了明确的解释：

- 消极自由：每位临床医生决定每个治疗过程的自主权；
- 积极自由：在一项专业中能够决定其成员应该具有多大程度的消极自由。

很多支持消极自由的人没有意识到，维护"积极自由"其实更有利。专业组织机构需要引领标准化的临床实践，或维护消极自由，否则，为了捍卫消极自由，他们将牺牲积极自由，而积极自由是最重要的。

照护路径的引入方式可以降低某些阻力。例如，当使用医学地图本土化一条路径时，应重点强调其适用于本地人口。路径的一些内容尚待本土化，如当地主要照护机构的名称及联系方式。有些内容不能改变，比如有充分证据和国家指南支持的药品处方。然而，在这个照护路径中，经常有一些步骤因为一些当地的情况而发生改变。例如，给患者提供参与随机对照试验的机会。

■ The inevitability of networking

Manuel Castells, one of the intellectual giants of the last 50 years, describes how networks are driving what he calls the Third Industrial Revolution(11). Castells cites the three drivers of this revolution as citizens, knowledge, and the Internet. Following technological developments over the last five years, it is now possible to substitute the smartphone for the Internet. Although Castells' analysis does not include healthcare, it is highly relevant to the development of health services in the 21st century. In this context, the driving forces in organisational development are patients, knowledge and the Internet, all of which interact with one another.

The Internet, by its very nature, promotes networks. It is not merely a passive transmitter of bits of information; it facilitates the creation of knowledge, for example, within healthcare, by allowing instant feedback from patients. The Internet helps to create what has been called a networked information economy.

The fundamental elements of the difference between the networked information economy and the mass media are network architecture and the cost of becoming a speaker. The first element is the shift from a hub-and-spoke architecture with unidirectional links to the end points in the mass media, to distributed architecture with multidirectional connections among all nodes in the networked information environment.(12)

■ The network as a complex adaptive system

The network will be the dominant type of organisation in the 21st century. In part this is due to the Internet, but it is also due to the recognition that the bureaucracy and the market, dominant types of organisation of the 20th century, have severe limitations. Networks have been referred to as complex adaptive systems: flexible, resilient and evolving, the best example of which is an ant colony(13).

To function as a complex adaptive system, a health service network requires the different types of clinician, who are clear about their respective roles within the network and their responsibilities towards the population served, to work together to increase value for the whole population.

■ Questions for reflection or for use in teaching or network building

If using these questions in network building or teaching, put one of the questions to the group and ask them to work in pairs to reflect on the question for three minutes; try to get people who do not know one another to work together. When taking feed-

■ 建立医疗卫生工作网络的必然性

曼纽尔·卡斯特是过去50年的科学巨人之一，他描述了工作网络是如何驱动了他所谓的"第三次工业革命"[11]。卡斯特认为：公民、知识和互联网是这次革命的3项驱动因素。过去5年随着技术的进步，智能手机代替互联网已经成为可能。尽管卡斯特的分析不包括医疗卫生领域，但该革命同21世纪医疗卫生服务的发展密切相关。在这一背景下，医疗卫生服务机构发展的驱动力就是患者、知识和互联网，且它们彼此相互影响。

互联网本身的特性是促进网络发展。它不仅是信息的被动传播载体，还能促进知识的产生：如在卫生保健领域，可以得到患者的即时反馈。互联网有助于带动所谓的网络信息经济。

网络信息经济与大众传媒的一些根本区别在于网络结构和成为一名演讲者的成本。网络结构从以前的单向连接到大众媒体终点的中心辐射结构，转变为网络信息环境中所有节点之间的多向连接的分布式结构。[12]

■ 工作网络是一个复杂的自适应系统

工作网络将会成为21世纪组织的主要运作形式。这在一定程度上要归功于互联网的发展，但也与人们认识到官僚机构和市场这两种20世纪占主导地位的组织形式均存在严重局限性有关。工作网络被认为是复杂的自适应系统，它具有灵活、适应性强且可不断调整完善的特点。其中蚁群就是最好的例子[13]。

要让这个复杂适应系统发挥功效，提供医疗服务的工作网络需要有不同类型的临床医生的共同参与。这些临床医生要明确自己在工作网络中的角色和对所服务人群的责任，才能共同为整个人群创造价值。

■ 互动思考题

如果在工作网络建设或教学中使用以下问题，可以将其中一个问题交给小组，让他们两人一组，思考3分钟，并尽量让彼此不认识的人一起工作。要求每组只能提出一个观点作为反馈。为了公平起见，让房间

back, let each pair make only one point. In the interests of equity, start with the pair on the left-hand side of the room for responses to the first question, then go to the pair on the right-hand side of the room for responses to the second question.

- Think of the best clinical network you know and list at least three of the network's characteristics that might explain its success;
- Think of a clinical network you know that does not work well and list at least three of the network's characteristics that might explain its poor performance;
- Imagine you are the Chief Executive of a hospital: what would be your main concerns about the involvement of 'your' clinicians in clinical networks?

References

(1) Child, J. (2005) Organization. Contemporary Principles and Practice. Blackwell Publishing. (p.15).

(2) Perrow, C. (1970) Organizational Analysis: a sociological view. Tavistock Publications, London.

(3) Wright, A. (2007) Glut. Mastering information through the ages. Joseph Henry Press, Washington DC. (p.7).

(4) Nelson, E.C., Batalden, P.B. and Godfrey, M.M. (2007) Quality by Design－A Clinical Microsystems Approach. John Wiley and Sons.

(5) Royal College of Paediatrics and Child Health (2006) A guide to understanding pathways and implementing networks. (p.9).

(6) McLellan, M., McKethan, A.N., Lewis, J.L., Roski, J., Fisher, E.S. (2010) A National Strategy to put Accountable Care Into Practice. Health Affairs 29 (5): 982.

左侧的一组开始回答第1个问题，然后让房间右侧的一组开始回答第2个问题。

- 回想你所知的最好的临床工作网络，并列举至少3个令其成功的特点；

- 回想你所知的效果不佳的临床工作网络，并列举至少3个令其表现不佳的特点；

- 如果你是一个医院的首席执行官：让手下临床医生融入到临床工作网络时，你最关注的问题是什么？

参 考 文 献

(7) Gray, J.A.M. (2009) Evidence-Based Healthcare. Churchill Livingstone.

(8) NHS Scotland (2008) A Workbook for People Starting to Develop Integrated Care Pathways.

(9) Timmermans, S. and Berg, M. (2003) The Gold Standard. The challenge of evidence-based medicine and standardization in health care. Temple University Press, Philadelphia (p.53).

(10) Berlin, I. (1958) Two Concepts of Liberty, in Four Essays on Liberty.

(11) Castells, M. (2004) The Network Society. Edward Elgar.

(12) Benkler, Y. (2006) The Wealth of Networks. How social production transforms markets and freedom. Yale University Press, New Haven and London (p.212).

(13) Holldobler, B. and Wilson, E.O. (1990) The Ants. Springer.

Chapter 8
ENGAGING PATIENTS

第八章
患者参与

This chapter will:

- describe the benefits and importance of patient engagement;
- analyse different ways in which engagement can improve the quality and increase the value of healthcare;
- describe the importance and duel role of patients' organisations.

By the end of this chapter, you will have developed an understanding of:

- the importance of patient engagement in health service development and delivery;
- how patient engagement can inform the debate about resource allocation and resource constraints;
- how patients' organisations can be supported.

■ What's in a name: patients or principals?

'Patients, customers, consumers, clients?We just call them punters. Let's face it, you are taking a chance every time you come into healthcare.'
—Doctor in Belfast

Patient: there is a move away from using this term; many professionals prefer to use 'citizen'. Alternatively, some professionals prefer to use terms such as 'people with diabetes' rather than 'diabetic patients' to ensure that a person is not characterised by their condition. In this chapter, the term 'patients' will be used as shorthand for people who have, or fear they have, a condition that could be helped by clinical intervention.

Principal: Economists often describe doctors as 'agents' because they act on behalf of the patient. The doctor (agent) is informed about a patient's health and their treatment options. The patient (principal) is relatively uninformed about these matters and therefore has to rely on the doctor to act in their (the patient's) best interests. A person will employ the services of an agent if they believe that their utility afterwards will be greater than without the help of the agent.(1)

From a legal perspective also, the patient is the principal, and the professional is the agent.

本章涉及内容：

● 描述患者参与的益处和重要性；

● 分析患者参与提升医疗卫生质量和价值的不同方式；

● 描述患者组织的重要性和双重角色。

在本章末，读者将会深入理解：

● 患者参与卫生事业发展和供给的重要性；

● 患者参与在资源分配和资源限制的讨论中所起到的作用；

● 如何支持患者组织。

■ 我们该如何定位所服务的人？将其视为患者还是委托人？

患者、顾客、消费者、客户？我们只把他们称之为投注者。直面现实吧，他们每次就诊时，都是经历一次博弈。

——来自贝尔法斯特的医生

患者：当前正倾向于避免使用这一词汇，许多专业人士倾向于称之为"公民"。或者，一些专业人士偏好使用"患糖尿病的人"而非"糖尿病患者"，以避免用疾病来定义患者。在本章节，"患者"这个词被用于代指：患有或可能患有通过医学干预可缓解的疾病的人。

委托人：医生代表患者行事，因此经济学家经常将他们描述为"代理人"。医生（代理人）知晓患者的健康状况及治疗选择方案，而患者（委托人）对此反而相对了解较少，因此不得不依靠医生为自己（患者）的最大利益行事。一个人雇佣代理人是相信在该代理人的帮助下，自己能获得更大利益。[1]

从法律角度讲亦然，患者是委托方，而医疗专业人士则是代理人。

■ The new healthcare paradigm

Systems of care offer a new paradigm for healthcare in the 21st century. One of the changes brought in with this new paradigm is a shift from doctor-centred to patient-centred care. If the 20th century was the century of the clinician, the 21st century will be the century of the patient. This shift is one of the most important aspects of the change in paradigm that is currently taking place (see Figure 8.1).

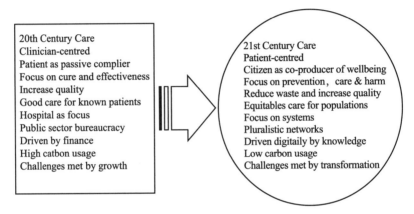

Figure 8.1 The new healthcare paradigm for the 21st century

The implications of this shift are important for all clinicians irrespective of their different roles in relation to the population served, including:

- *caring for individual patients*;
- *managing a service*;
- *taking responsibility for the whole population of patients*.

All clinicians need to adopt a new approach towards patients and understand the benefits that engaging patients will bring. Although one approach is to treat patients as equals in the healthcare transaction, this would not be sufficient because it is now accepted that patients have a major contribution to make to the development and delivery of health services.

■ 新型的医疗卫生范式

21世纪医疗系统迎来了新型医疗卫生范式。这种新范式带来的改变之一，是医疗从原来的以医生为中心转变为以患者为中心。如果说20世纪的医疗范式是以医生为中心的，那么21世纪将是以患者为中心。这是当前的医疗范式最重要的转变之一（图8.1）。

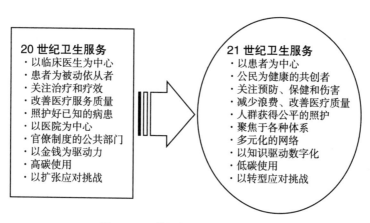

图8.1　21世纪新型医疗卫生范式

不管临床医生在服务的人群中扮演着何种角色，这种以患者为中心的医疗范式的变化对所有临床医生来说都很重要。这种新范式需要：

● 照护个体患者；

● 管理医疗服务；

● 为患病人群负责。

所有临床医生都需要采用新方式对待患者，并理解患者的参与会给医疗带来的益处。尽管其中的一种方式是在医疗过程中将患者放在与自己平等的位置上，但这还不够，因为现在普遍认为患者在医疗卫生保健的发展和实践的过程中都至关重要。

■ The benefits of engaging patients

The main outcome of engaging patients is what is known as 'coproduction'.

Co-production means delivering public services in an equal and recipro-cal relationship between professionals, people using services, their families and their neighbours. Where activities are co-produced in this way, both services and neighbourhoods become far more effective agents of change. (2)

Co-production can confer benefit in three domains of health service management:
- *engagement for performance improvement;*
- *engagement in decision-making;*
- *engagement to increase value.*

Presenting these domains as a list does not show the potential for interaction and synergy, which is best conveyed diagrammatically (see Figure 8.2).

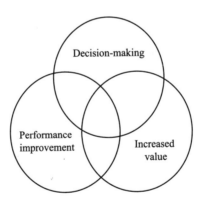

Figure 8.2 The three domains of health service management that benefit from patient engagement

■ Rules of engagement

- *The clinician responsible for the management of a clinical service has to relate to the patients currently in contact with that service.*
- *The clinician responsible for population healthcare has to relate to all people in need, irrespective of whether they have been referred or are in contact with the service.*

■ 患者参与的益处

患者参与的主要结果就是所谓的"医患共为"。

"医患共为"指的是在医务工作者、医疗卫生保健使用者及其家人和邻里之间以平等互惠的关系提供医疗卫生。在那些以"医患共为"方式开展活动的地方，医疗卫生供给和相应社区都会成为更有效的变革推动者。[2]

"医患共为"能在医疗卫生管理方面带来以下3个好处：

- 参与绩效提升；
- 参与决策；
- 参与价值提高。

单纯的文字罗列不能体现三者之间交互协同的潜质，用图表的形式则可以很好地体现（图8.2）。

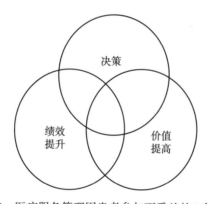

图8.2 医疗服务管理因患者参与而受益的3个方面

■ 参与规则

- 负责管理某项临床干预的医生必须从目前接触该项目的患者的角度考虑问题；
- 践行群医学的医生，必须考虑到所有有需要的人，无论是已被转诊者还是接受治疗者。

■ Engaging the patients seen by a clinical service

Throughout the book we have emphasized the difference in managerial accountability for a service, that is to the patients using the service and accountability to a population, some of whose members may be direct users of the service, with others being supported indirectly. This book focuses on the latter responsibility, on population medicine but it is essential to use any opportunities to engage with patients. Engagement with people who are users of a specialist service reaches one part of the population and although it is insufficient by itself as a means of engaging with the whole population in need its potential should be realized by activities such as.

- *Ensuring a patient or care representative on planning and development groups;*
- *Getting feedback from patients, for example by using www. iwantgreat-care. org or simple suggestion boxes;*
- *Supporting the local branch of the relevant national charity.*

This is happening in many services and health centres at present but what is not happening is the engagement of people in need who are not yet being cared for by the service. There is a need to engage with the whole population.

■ Engaging with all the patients in the population

It is common to find that the patients being seen by a specialist service are not necessarily those who would benefit most from the service (see Figure 8.3).

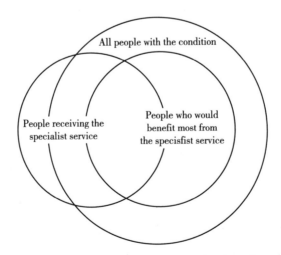

Figure 8.3 The relationship between need and service use

■ 使接受临床服务的患者参与其中

在整本书中，我们一直在强调医疗服务的两种管理职责之间的区别：一种是针对使用服务的患者；另一种是针对人群，该群体中一部分可能是直接使用者，而对其他人则是间接的提供支持。本书关注的是后一种职责——群医学，有必要利用一切机会让患者参与其中。与专科医疗的就诊者建立关联，让总人口中一部分人群得到了照护。尽管这种方式还不能囊括整个有需求的群体，不过其潜力可通过以下活动表现出来：

- 确保在医疗规划和发展团队中有患者或照护者的代表；
- 获取患者的反馈，例如使用www.iwantgreatcare.org或提供意见箱；
- 支持国家相关慈善机构的地方分支机构。

虽然在许多医疗卫生服务中心都在进行这些活动，但那些有需求却没获得医疗照护的人还没有参与其中。让整个有需要的群体都参与进来，这一点非常重要。

■ 让人群中所有患者都参与其中

我们经常会发现，接受专科医疗服务的那些患者并不一定是从中受益最多的人（图8.3）。

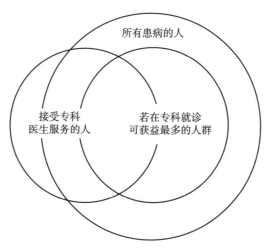

图8.3 医疗服务需求与利用之间的关系

One response to this phenomenon is to increase the size of the specialist service; however, this may not be possible in an era of zero growth. Even if increased resources are available, simply providing more of the same would not maximise value. Instead, action needs to be taken:

- *To ensure that those people who will benefit most from specialist care are referred, for example, by providing training and guidelines to generalist clinicians for example, domiciliary nurses, community pharmacists and general practitioners;*
- *To increase the knowledge, skill and confidence of all clinicians treating the population so that generalists are able to care for a greater range of patients without referral to specialists; this requires the provision of not only training but also the type of support that can be given easily by telephone and email.*

As emphasised in Chapter 2, this approach will increase value from the resources available. It is also an expression of a new culture in which all healthcare professionals, generalists and specialists, work together to care for all the patients with a particular problem. The drawback is that this is a one-way process, from clinician to patient.

To complement the feedback that individual patients are able to give, either about the consultation they have just had or about the service as a whole, is the development of a working relationship between all clinicians and all patients and carers in the population, most easily through the relevant patients' organisations. Many patients' organisations already undertake a dual function (see Figure 8.4):

1. lobbying the body responsible for resource allocation for increased resources for their particular community of patients;

2. helping the relevant service directly, not only by raising funds but also by providing peer-support for newly diagnosed patients and information for patients and carers.

　　一种应对这种现象的措施是提高专科医疗服务的规模，但是这种应对方式在医疗资源零增长的时代不太可行。即使医疗资源能有所增加，仅靠提供更多相同类型的医疗服务仍不能实现价值的最大化。因此我们应该采取以下措施：

- 确保从专科医疗服务中受益最多的人被转诊到专科：例如，通过对全科工作者——家庭护士、社区药剂师、全科医生等——提供培训和指南来实现；
- 所有对人群服务的医务人员都应丰富知识、增长技能和提高信心。这样就可使全科工作者能为更多患者提供医疗服务而无须把这些患者转诊至专科。这不仅需要为医务人员提供培训，还可采用更简易可行方法如通过电话和电子邮件等给予帮助。

　　如本书第二章中所强调的，此类举措可以提高现有可用资源的价值，也展现了一种新的医疗文化：即所有的医务人员、全科工作者和专科医生，一起为有特定医疗需求的患者提供服务。然而缺点是此过程是从医生到患者的单向过程。

　　补充患者的反馈意见——无论是对于刚结束的问诊还是对于整体服务评价——就能让人群中的所有临床医生、患者和护理人员建立工作关系。这最容易通过相关患者组织来实现。很多患者组织已经起到了类似的双重作用（图8.4）：

1. 游说负责医疗资源分配的部门，为特定的患者群体增加医疗资源；
2. 为相关的服务提供直接的帮助，不仅是筹集资金，而且还为新确诊的患者提供同伴支持，并为患者和照护者提供相关信息。

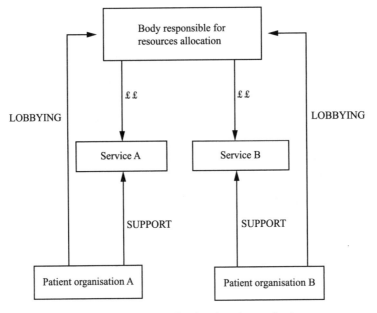

Figure 8.4 The dual role of patients' organisations

■ Supporting patients' organisations

The clinician practising population medicine can engage with patients other than those in direct contact with the specialist service by supporting the relevant patient organisation (see Box 8.1). Just as the individual patient is a partner in their care, the community of patients is a partner in the network that delivers services to them.

Box 8.1 Ways in which clinicians practising population medicine
can engage with patient organisations

- If a local branch of a patient organisation does not exist, ask the relevant national patient organisation to set one up
- Offer the local patients' organisation practical help, for example, by providing rooms for local meetings
- Offer to attend local meetings to ensure the organisation obtains best current knowledge about evidence from the published literature and about the services provided
- Participate in fundraising events for the organisation

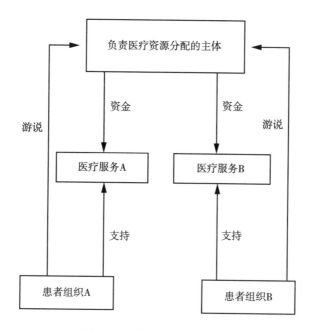

图8.4 患者组织的双重作用

■ 支持患者组织

践行群医学的临床医生可以通过支持相关的患者组织，让所有患者参与进来，而非仅限于那些来专科就诊的患者（专栏8.1）。正如患者个体是其医疗过程中的参与者，患者组织也是医疗服务实施网络中的一部分。

专栏8.1 践行群医学的临床医生让患者组织参与进来的方法

- 如果当地没有患者组织的分支机构，则要求相关的国家级患者组织在当地建立一个分支机构；
- 向当地患者组织提供实际帮助，如为举办会议提供场所；
- 主动参加当地的会议，以确保患者组织能在已出版的文献中获取有关证据的最新知识以及所提供医疗卫生的最新信息；
- 参加经费募集活动。

■ Engaging the public

As resource allocation decisions are concerned with equity, or fairness, rather than efficiency (3), it is important to engage with the population paying for healthcare when making them. There are two main types of resource allocation in which the public may become engaged during decision-making about service provision:

1. The allocation of resources within a service or programme, which is the responsibility of clinicians and managers within each service who must engage with the patients who use that service and their representatives;

2. The allocation of resources across services or programmes, which is the responsibility of those who pay for healthcare or, in NHS England, commissioners, who must engage with the public as well as patients and their representatives.

Although a patient organisation is focused on winning increased resources for the service or programme relevant to their members, it will have implications for other services. Similarly, there may be strong public reaction against proposed change to an individual service, such as the closure of a small but important paediatric service, even when the key healthcare professionals involved are in favour of the change; however, if the service is not closed, there is likely to be a negative impact on other services at the hospital.

If the public are not involved in the whole debate about resource allocation, the focus for argument may fall on one particular 'priority' after another, leading to demands that each should be funded, in the absence of a public appreciation that in allocating resources for one purpose there is an opportunity cost through which resources are denied to another group of patients.

By involving the public, and by definition their political representatives, in the debate and decision-making, payers are able to shift the focus from being held to account for meeting every need to being held to account for the reasonableness of their decision-making (4) (see Chapter 1).

■ Questions for reflection or for use in teaching or network building

If using these questions in network building or teaching, put one of the questions to the group and ask them to work in pairs to reflect on the question for three minutes; try to get people who do not know one another to work together. When taking feedback, let each pair make only one point. In the interests of equity, start with the pair on

■ 让公众参与其中

医疗资源配置决策关注的是平等或公平，而不仅是效率[3]。因此在制定这些决策时，让那些为医疗卫生付费的群体参与其中是非常重要的。在有公众参与的医疗服务决策过程中，主要有两种医疗资源分配类型：

1. 对某一医疗卫生服务或项目的内部资源分配，是实施此项医疗卫生的医务人员和管理者的责任。他们必须让接受这项服务的患者及代表都参与其中；

2. 对医疗卫生服务或项目之间进行资源分配，是医疗卫生付费方的责任，或者在NHS中，是专员的责任，他们必须让公众、患者及其代表接触。

尽管患者组织总是会努力为与他们的成员相关的医疗服务或项目争取获得更多资源，但这也会对其他服务产生影响。与此类似，当提议改革某项医疗服务时（如关闭某项小却重要的儿科服务），可能会遭到公众强烈反对，即使医疗卫生界重要人士对此投赞成票。然而，如果这项服务不关闭，则将可能对医院的其他服务产生负面影响。

如果公众不能参与医疗资源分配的讨论，则争论焦点就会落在一个又一个特定的"优先"项目上，从而出现认为每个"优先"项目都应该得到资金支持的呼声。如果公众没有意识到，在为一个目的分配资源时，存在一种机会成本，其结果是另一个患者群体无法得到资源。

通过让公众及其所指定的政治代表能参与讨论和决策，为医疗卫生付费的人们就能将关注点从满足每项需求转到关注其决策的合理性上来[4]（见第1章）。

■ 互动思考题

如果在工作网络建设或教学中使用以下问题，可以将其中一个问题交给小组，让他们两人一组，思考3分钟，并尽量让彼此不认识的人一起工作。要求每组只能提出一个观点作为反馈。为了公平起见，让房间

the left-hand side of the room for responses to the first question, then go to the pair on the right-hand side of the room for responses to the second question.

- What are the disadvantages of engaging patients and their representatives in the management of services?
- What three points would you emphasise when making a presentation to a group of sceptical clinicians about increased engagement of patients;
- A patient group has nominated somebody to be their representative on a management team. They ask you for guidance about the duties of a 'patient representative' in this situation. Identify five points about the responsibilities this role would involve.

References

(1) Wonderling, D., Gruen, R. and Black, N. (2005) Introduction to Health Economics. Understanding Public Health. Open University Press (p.100).

(2) Boyle, D. and Harris M. (2009) Discussion Paper: The Challenge of Co-Production. How equal partnerships between professionals and the public are crucial to improving public services. NESTA (p.11).

左侧的一组开始回答第1个问题，然后让房间右侧的一组开始回答第2个问题。

- 让患者及其代表参与医疗管理时，会有哪些弊端？
- 当你给那些对提高患者参与度持怀疑态度的医生作报告时，你会强调哪3点？
- 一个患者团体已经提名了某人担任其管理团队的代表，他们向你寻求关于这种情况下"患者代表"的职责指导，请给出这个角色责任的五个要点。

参考文献

（3）Anand, S.（2004）The Concern for Equity in Health. In: Anand, S., Peter, F. and Sen, A.（Eds）. Public Health, Ethics and Equity. Oxford University Press（p.15）.

（4）Daniels, N. and Sabin, J.E.（2008）Setting Limits Fairly, Learning to Share Resources for Health. Oxford University Press（p.44）.

Chapter 9
CREATING BUDGETS FOR POPULATIONS

第九章
为人群编制预算

This chapter will:

- discuss how programme budgeting provides a context to encourage dission-making to maximise value;
- describe how to build a budget even if the finance is in different parts of the health service;
- describe how to create a budget even if the financial data are not available.

By the end of the chapter, you will have developed an understanding of:

- all the resources that need to be included in a programme or system budget;
- steps that can be taken to increase value;
- rules of thumb for estimating spend even when no financial data are available.

Budget: The contents of a bag or wallet...A statement of the probable revenue and expenditure for the forthcoming year.

—*Shorter Oxford English Dictionary*

The meaning of the term 'a budget' includes other resources in addition to financial resources. A budget is not a synonym for healthcare finance. Thus, the resources available to a clinician practicing population medicine are greater than the financial resources of the service for which they may be managerially responsible because the potential resources include the contributions of volunteers, carers and patients (see Figure 9.1).

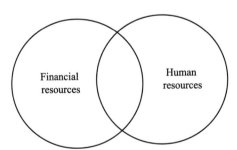

Figure 9.1 The resources of healthcare

本章涉及内容：

- 讨论项目预算编制如何为鼓励决策价值最大化提供背景；
- 描述如果财政资源分布在医疗卫生服务的不同部门时，该如何编制预算；
- 描述即使在无法获得财务数据的情况下，该如何编制预算。

在本章末，读者将会深入理解：

- 项目预算或系统预算需包括的资源；
- 增加价值应采取的步骤；
- 在没有财务数据的情况下估计支出的经验法则。

预算：袋子里或钱包里的东西……下一年可能的收入和支出报表。

——《简明牛津英语字典》

"预算"一词的含义也包括除财务资源外的其他资源。预算并不是医疗筹资的代名词。因此，从事群医学的临床医生可利用的资源往往多于机构的财务资源，还有可能来自于志愿者、医疗卫生人员和患者的贡献（图9.1）。

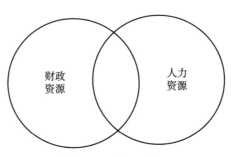

图9.1　医疗卫生资源

It is important for clinicians practising population medicine to be good stewards of all resources irrespective of whether the resources they are responsible for committing are directly charged to their budget (see Figure 9.2). Types of expenditure that tend not to be directly charged to clinical budgets include laboratory tests or imaging.

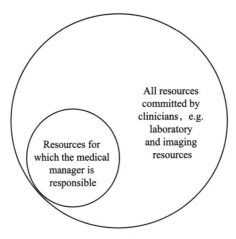

Figure 9.2 Direct and indirect responsibility for resources in a health service

■ Leadership and budget management

The creation of population healthcare is a leadership and not a managerial task. It is primarily concerned with culture change and not bureaucratic control. The key considerations for clinicians responsible for systems of care are:

1. the population they serve, not just the patients referred;

2. the need to be good stewards of all the resources already available before they bid for increased resources;

3. the need to be part of a community of practice, all of whose members and their resources need to be treated with respect and altruism.

Medical managers usually have responsibility for, and authority over, a delegated budget. As shown in Figures 9.1 and 9.2, clinicians with responsibility for a population need to mobilise both financial and human resources over which they have no direct managerial control. Indeed, such clinicians may not have control over the financial resources for the specialist service in which they work. This is because the role of the clinician with responsibility to and for a population will usually be different from that of departmental manager, particularly if both roles include clinical responsibilities.

对于践行群医学的临床医生来说，重要的是做好所有资源的统筹管理，无论他们所负责的资源是否直接纳入预算（图9.2）。通常未直接纳入临床预算的支出类型包括实验室检验或影像学检查。

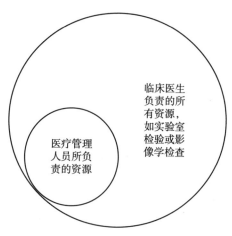

图9.2 医疗卫生服务资源的直接与间接责任

■领导力和预算管理

群医学中的创新行动是领导力的体现，而非一项管理任务。它主要关注的是文化转变，而非行政管控。负责医疗卫生系统的临床医生应考虑的关键因素有：

1. 他们负责的人群，而不只是转诊来的患者；

2. 在争取到新增资源之前需要管理好所有可用资源；

3. 需要成为社区卫生工作中的一员，尊重社区中所有成员和资源并遵守"利他"原则。

医疗管理者通常有责任也有权力管理划拨预算。如图9.1和图9.2所示，负责某个人群的临床医生还需要调动不由自己直接管控的财务和人力资源。事实上，这些临床医生可能无法控制他们所在专科的财政资源。这是因为对人群负责的临床医生的角色通常与部门管理者的角色是不同的，特别是当这两个角色都肩负临床责任时。

The clinician with responsibility for a population has to mobilise the required resources through leadership rather than management: managers are responsible for the day-to-day operation of a service, whereas the leaders are primarily responsible for shaping the culture. The culture needed to promote population healthcare is shown in Box 9.1. The culture for population healthcare is not the type of command-and-control culture that evolves when a single department or institution pursues a particular target.

Although it has been popular for the last few decades, there is increasing evidence that the approach of pressing people to perform well and rewarding them financially if they do so is not only less effective than was originally thought but also has severe adverse effects (1, 2). Furthermore, a culture in which institutions compete with one another for prestige, power and money results in behaviour by which other services are exploited or even deceived.

The model for population healthcare is that of a complex adaptive system, the best example of which is the ant colony. Ants do not compete at the level of the individual: the whole colony works together and different groups of ant within the colony cooperate and make sacrifices for the benefit of the whole. Promoting a culture supportive of population healthcare represents a leadership challenge especially when trying to make the best use of programme or system budgets.

Box 9.1 The culture of population healthcare

- All the agencies involved are focused on the population to be served, not their own well-being
- People in one organisation are concerned about possible adverse effects of decisions on other organisations and seek to mitigate them
- Individuals and individual organisations behave altruistically, that is, they may take decisions or behave in ways that are not advantageous to their particular position in the short term

■ Programme budgets

A programme consists of a set of systems with a common knowledge base and a common budget. Programme budgeting is a technique that enables personnel in a health service to identify how much money has been invested in major health programmes, with a view to making future investment decisions more rational and have a greater focus on value.

While the terms 'budgeting' and 'budgets' are normally applied to current and/or future allocations of expenditure, in the context of programme budgeting and programme budgets, it is assumed that they can be applied to past alloca-

负责人群的临床医生必须通过领导力而非管理来调动所需的资源：管理者负责工作的日常运营，而领导者主要负责塑造文化。促进群医学实践所需的文化见专栏9.1。群医学的文化并非那种由单个部门或机构追求特定目标演化而来的指挥−控制文化。

尽管这在过去的几十年里很流行，但越来越多的证据表明，为激励人们努力工作所设定经济上的奖励机制，不仅不像最初认为的那样有效，还会产生严重的负面影响[1, 2]。此外，各机构为了威望、权力和金钱而相互竞争的文化，会导致服务被过度使用甚至错误应用。

群医学的模型是一个复杂的自适应系统，其中最好的例子是蚁群。蚂蚁不在个体层面上竞争：整个蚁群一起工作，蚁群内不同的小组为了整体的利益互相合作和做出牺牲。推动有利于群医学的文化的形成是对领导力的挑战，特别是在试图最佳地利用项目或系统的预算时。

专栏9.1 群医学文化

- 所有相关机构所关注的是其服务的人群而非自身的福祉。
- 在一个组织中，人们所关心的是自己的决策是否会给其他组织带来的不利影响并想方设法减轻这些影响。
- 个人和各个组织的行为是利他的，也就是说，他们可能做出在短期内对自己特定地位不利的决定或行为。

■ 项目预算

项目由一套具有共同知识库和共同预算的系统组成。编制项目预算是一门技术活，可使医疗卫生人员明确在重大医疗卫生项目中投入了多少资金，以期今后的投资决策更加合理并更注重价值。

虽然"预算编制"和"预算"一词通常适用于目前和/或未来的支出分配，但在项目预算编制和项目预算的语境中，它们也可用于过去的款项配置。项目预算编制的潜在基本原则非常简单。如果依据宽泛的医疗卫生目标和优先项目做出决定，那么提供的数据的广泛程度应该与各项选择相匹配。例如

tions as well. The principle underlying programme budgeting is very simple. If decisions are to be made about broadly defined health — care objectives and priorities — for example, what are the objectives associated with care of the elderly? What relative priorities are attached to the treatment of cancer compared with the prevention of heart disease? — then data should be provided in similarly broad terms to match the nature of the choices. (3)

The NHS in England is fortunate because it has one of the best national programme budget schemes in the world, first initiated in 2002. At the time of writing, there are 23 programme budgets in NHS England, based on the World Health Organization's International Classification of Diseases 10 (ICD10). This information provides the NHS with an opportunity unique among countries with developed economies to identify:

- *where resources are currently being invested*;
- *the value of those investments by relating outcomes to resources*;
- *the most effective way of investing in health services in future in relation to the needs of the population.*

Estimated expenditure for 2010/11 on each programme in NHS England is set out in Table 9.1. The advantages of programme budgeting are:

- *the potential to engage clinicians in discussions about value for money when conventional budgetary procedures have failed*;
- *increased involvement of clinicians in resource allocation*;
- *improved information support during decision-making by payers for or commissioners of healthcare*;
- *the potential to involve the public and patients in decisions about resource allocation.*

"照护老年人的目标是什么？与预防心脏病相比，癌症治疗方面有哪些相对优先事项？"。[3]

NHS幸运地拥有世界上最好的国家项目预算方案之一。该方案制定于2002年。在撰写本书时，根据世界卫生组织的国际疾病分类第10次修订本（ICD10），NHS已有23个项目预算。这些信息为NHS提供了一个在发达国家中独一无二的机会来明确以下问题：

● 目前正在哪里投入资源；

● 将资源与结局挂钩后的投资价值；

● 根据人口的需要，对未来医疗卫生进行投资的最有效方式。

表9.1列出了2010/2011年度NHS各项目的预算开支。项目预算的优点有：

● 当常规预算程序未得到有效执行时，可让临床医生参与投资价值的讨论；

● 提升临床医生对资源分配工作的参与度；

● 加强医疗卫生支付者或医疗卫生专员在决策过程中的信息支持；

● 为公众和患者参与资源分配决策创造条件。

Table 9.1 Programme budgeting estimated England-level gross expenditure for programmes in 2010/2011[①]

Programme budgeting category code	Programme budgeting category	Gross expenditure 2010/2011 (£ billion)
1	Infectious Diseases	1.80
2	Cancers & Tumours	5.81
3	Disorders of the Blood	1.36
4	Endocrine, Nutritional and Metabolic Problems	3.00
5	Mental Health Disorders	11.91
6	Problems of Learning Disability	2.90
7	Neurological	4.30
8	Problems of Vision	2.14
9	Problems of Hearing	0.45
10	Problems of Circulation	7.72
11	Problems of the Respiratory System	4.43
12	Dental Problems	3.31
13	Problems of the Gastro-Intestinal System	4.43
14	Problems of the Skin	2.13
15	Problems of the Musculo-Skeletal System	5.06
16	Problems due to Trauma and Injuries	3.75
17	Problems of the Genito-Urinary System	4.78
18	Maternity and Reproductive Health	3.44
19	Conditions of Neonates	1.05
20	Adverse Effects and Poisoning	0.96
21	Healthy Individuals	2.15
22	Social Care Needs	4.18
23	Other Areas of Spend/Conditions	25.95
Total		107.00

There are, however, some weaknesses associated with programme budgeting in England (see Box 9.2).

① http://www.dh.gov.uk/health/2012/08/programme-budgeting-data/

表9.1 2010/2011年度英国医疗服务项目的总预算①

项目预算类别编号	项目预算类别	2010/2011年度总支出 （亿英镑）
1	感染性疾病	18.0
2	癌症和肿瘤	58.1
3	血液疾病	13.6
4	内分泌、营养和代谢疾病	30.0
5	精神健康障碍	119.1
6	学习障碍	29.0
7	神经系统疾病	43.0
8	视力障碍	21.4
9	听力障碍	4.5
10	循环系统疾病	77.2
11	呼吸系统疾病	44.3
12	口腔疾病	33.1
13	消化系统疾病	44.3
14	皮肤病	21.3
15	肌肉-骨骼系统疾病	50.6
16	外伤和创伤疾病	37.5
17	泌尿生殖系统疾病	47.8
18	产妇和生殖健康	34.4
19	新生儿健康	10.5
20	不良反应和中毒	9.6
21	个体健康	21.5
22	社会关怀需求	41.8
23	其他领域的支出/问题	259.5
合计		1070.0

然而，英国的项目预算仍有一些缺点（专栏9.2）。

---

① http://www.dh.gov.uk/health/2012/08/programme-budgeting-data/

Despite the weaknesses inherent in the programme budgeting scheme for NHS England, the data are very useful. Programme budgeting information enables the clinician responsible for population medicine to improve healthcare for the local population. To ensure the usefulness of the data, however, they need to be:

- *reproduced at the level at which resources are actually allocated, for example, in a county like Derbyshire, with a population of 600,000, as well as at national level;*
- *related to outcome;*
- *owned by the clinicians who commit the resources;*
- *further subdivided by systems.*

Box 9.2 Weaknesses in the construction of national programme budgets in NHS England

- Although the cost of drugs prescribed in general practice and the cost of referrals made are assigned to relevant budgets, the cost of primary care professionals' time, principally that of general practitioners, is not assigned to the relevant budgets
- The category 'Other' represents spend not classified by disease programme, and is very large; included within this budget are primary care, education, and the costs of many of the bureaucratic bodies that run the NHS
- Expenditure on education, research and management is not assigned to relevant programme budgets
- Budgets are expressed only in financial terms; the 21.8 million tonnes of carbon produced by the NHS each year should be assigned to programme budgets in a similar way
- Some of the programme budgets have less granularity than others; for example, in the Cancers and Tumours budget, it is possible to identify the amount spent on each of the common cancers, whereas in the budget for Problems of the Respiratory System, although there are sub-budgets for asthma and chronic obstructive pulmonary disease (COPD), the biggest sub-budget is 'Other'; coding will improve as programme budgets grow in importance
- The underlying assumption for programme budgets is that people have a single diagnosis; however, as many people have more than one diagnosis, it is useful to base programme budgets on populations, such as frail elderly people, as well as on conditions (see Figure 9.3)

尽管NHS的项目预算存在一些固有的缺点，但其数据非常有用。项目预算信息可使群医学医生改善当地人群的医疗卫生状况。然而，为了充分利用数据，这些数据还需要：

- 在国家分配资源的基础上，结合当地实际情况，如拥有60万人口的德比郡，再进行预算；
- 与结局相关；
- 由负责统筹资源的临床医生拥有；
- 按系统进一步细分。

专栏9.2　NHS国家方案预算的缺点

- 虽然全科医生的处方药费和转诊费用划拨到相关预算中，但初级保健专业人员的时间成本，主要是全科医生的时间成本，没有划拨到相关预算中。
- "其他"类是指没有按疾病分类的支出，数额很大；这一预算包括初级保健、教育和许多运行NHS的政府机构的费用。
- 教育、研究和管理方面的支出未被划拨给相关的方案预算。
- 预算只以财务术语表示；NHS每年的2180万吨碳排放应该以类似的方式分配到项目预算中。
- 有些项目预算的细致度不如其他项目；例如，在癌症和肿瘤预算中，可以确定用于每一种常见癌症的金额，而在呼吸系统问题的预算中，尽管有用于哮喘和慢性阻塞性肺疾病的子预算，但最大的子预算出现在"其他"中；随着项目预算重要性的增加，编码工作将得到改善。
- 项目预算的潜在假设是人们只有单一的疾病诊断。然而，由于很多人被诊断患有一种以上的疾病，所以最好按人群来编制预算，如按年老体弱者和不同的情况（疾病）编制（图9.3）。

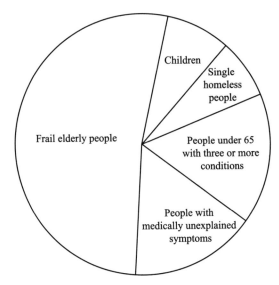

Figure 9.3 Population-based programmes of care

■ System-specific budgets

Whereas a programme is at the level of Cancers and Tumours, Mental Health Disorders or Problems of the Respiratory System, the system is at a finer level of granularity. To take respiratory health as an example, within that programme there are systems of care for asthma, chronic obstructive pulmonary disease (COPD), and sleep apnoea. Therefore, the person responsible for a population-based programme almost always has an additional responsibility for several popula-tion-based systems of care.

Furthermore, each of the systems within a programme may be championed by a clinician keen to develop the system for which they are responsible. Thus, the person responsible for a population-based programme not only has to compete with other programmes either to increase resources or to prevent resources being taken away, they also have to deal with competing claims from clinicians respon-sible for the systems of care within that programme (see Figure 9.4).

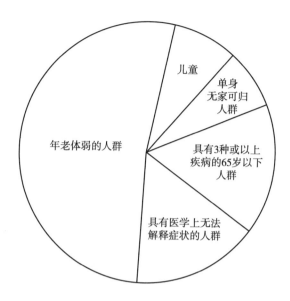

图9.3 以人群为基础的医疗项目

■子系统的特定预算

项目是建立在癌症和肿瘤、精神健康障碍或呼吸系统问题这样的层面上，而系统则是建立在更细化的层面。例如，在呼吸系统项目包括了哮喘、慢性阻塞性肺疾病和睡眠呼吸暂停综合征在内的多个医疗卫生系统。因此，一个以人群为基础的项目负责人，总是需要对多个以人群为基础的照护系统负有额外的责任。

此外，项目中的每一个子系统的牵头人都可能是热衷于建设自己负责部分的临床医生。因此，群医学的项目负责人不仅需要与其他项目竞争，引进资源或防止资源流失，还必须要处理好项目内部负责各医疗系统的医生之间相互竞争（图9.4）。

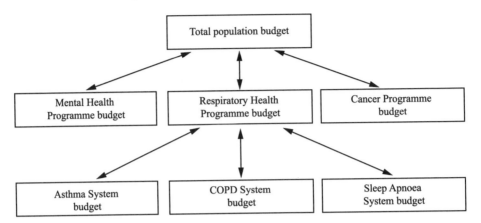

Figure 9.4 Programme and system budgets

People who commission or pay for healthcare must make decisions about the allocation of resources to different programmes, addressing questions such as:

- *Should we switch resources from one programme to another?*
- *Into which programme should we invest new resources?*
- *From which programme should we cut resources?*

Once the budget has been allocated to a programme, however, the clinician practising population medicine has to ask an analogous set of questions.

- *Have we got the distribution of resources right among the various systems of care within the programme or should we redistribute?*
- *If I have to make a cut from one of the services, which should it be?*
- *If I am able to release some resources, to which of the services should those resources be given?*

When practising population medicine, it is essential to be aware of all the key resources that are being spent on a particular condition or a group of conditions within the population served, irrespective of which institutions are responsible for the management of those resources. Rarely is a financial budget for a system available at a local level. Usually it has to be created using the framework in Table 9.2. The simplest approach is to prepare an inventory of all the key resources used, and once they have been listed to express the financial costs of those resources; if there are no accurate costings available, then it is important to make an estimate.

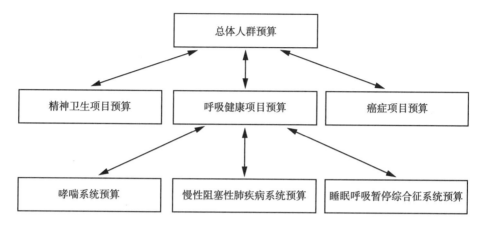

图9.4 项目与系统预算

医疗卫生的支付者或委托人必须决定不同项目之间的资源分配并解决以下问题：

- 我们应该把资源从一个项目转到另一个项目吗？
- 我们应该为哪个项目投入新资源？
- 我们应该从哪个项目削减资源？

若某个项目获得了预算，那么群医学医生必须考虑以下类似的问题：

- 资源是否已在项目内各照护系统之间正确分配，还是应该重新分配？
- 如果必须从中削减一项服务，应该削减哪一项？
- 如果我能够支配一些资源，那么这些资源应该分给哪些服务项目？

在践行群医学中，无论由哪个机构负责管理资源，都必须了解分配给特定疾病或特定患者人群的所有重要资源。一个仅限于当地的系统很少能得到财政预算。编制系统预算通常要依据表9.2的框架。最简单的方法就是准备一份清单，列明所使用的全部重要资源，财务成本也就随之明朗；若得不到准确的成本核算，那么进行估算也同样重要。

Sometimes, it is relatively easy to identify the financial spend and the use of resources on a specific condition if the service is discrete, but in some specialties clinicians will deal with more that one condition during the same clinic, and in primary care the general practitioner will deal with many conditions — from asthma to depression to heart failure to a medically unexplained symptom — during the course of one surgery. It should, however, be possible to estimate to the nearest million pounds what money is spent on a particular condition in a particular population. Estimates for services delivered to subgroups of that population, such as children or frail elderly people, are more difficult but should still be attempted.

The expenditure associated with calculating to the nearest pound the amount of money entailed in the delivery of a service is high. Any service in which an attempt is made to bill every item needs to spend a large amount on administration unless it is a specialist hospital doing only elective surgery on healthy people. The precise costing of a single episode of care, or the precise costing of a whole service, would not justify the level of expenditure on data collection except as a research exercise. Any service that has to deal with emergencies, or admits older people with four or more diagnoses, would face huge costs were it to try to account for every catheter or drip set. One of the joint winners of the Nobel Prize for Economics in 2009, Oliver Williamson, was recognized for his work over the last 20 years, which highlighted the large transaction costs associated with both markets and bureaucracies when they try to achieve greater efficiency through micromanagement.

■ Budget-building: key questions about key resources

The remainder of this chapter is dedicated to outlining the steps that can be taken to build a budget by mapping all the key resources, both human and financial, that are necessary for a system of care (see Table 9.2).

Building a budget, even if precise financial data are not available, is essential; it is better to be accurate than precise. Accuracy allows clinicians to focus their attention and use their clinical knowledge to obtain increased value from the resources available by asking the following questions, and answering them honestly.

- *Could we reallocate the resources among the services funded by the programme to achieve increased value for the common problems we face?*
- *Within the budget for each common problem, can we shift resources from lower-to higher-value interventions?*

有时，如果各类医疗照护互不相干，确定特定疾病的财务支出和资源利用还是相对容易的。然而，某些专科的临床医生会在同一诊所处理多种医疗问题；初级保健的全科医生会在一次应诊过程中处理多种疾病，如从哮喘到抑郁到心力衰竭再到医学上无法解释的症状。尽管如此，对特定人群特定疾病编制的经费估算应该可以精确到百万英镑；而对人群中某些群体（如儿童或年老体弱者）来说，编制医疗预算难度更大但仍需尝试进行。

计算医疗花费的精确数字本身就需要很高的成本。任何医疗机构在试图列出每一条账单细目时都需要耗费大量的管理资源，除非这所医院是一家特殊的专科医院，只为健康人做选择性手术。收集单项或整个医疗卫生的精确成本数据不能用来判断支出水平，除非是用于实验研究。若将收费精确到每一支导管或每一个输液装置，任何急诊或接诊患有4种及以上疾病老年人的医疗活动都将产生巨大开销。2009年诺贝尔经济学奖的共同获奖者之一奥利弗·威廉姆森因其过去20年的工作而得到认可。他的研究强调，市场和行政机构试图通过微观管理以获得更大效益时将会产生巨额交易成本。

■ 预算编制：与重要资源有关的关键问题

本章节剩余部分将通过绘制照护系统所需的所有关键资源（人力和财政资源）来概述制定预算所需的步骤（表9.2）。

即使得不到精确的财务数据，也有必要进行预算编制；预算的准确性比精确性更重要。准确的预算可以使临床医生集中注意力，运用自己的临床知识，通过提出并诚实地回答以下问题，从而从可用资源中获得更大价值。

● 我们能否重新分配项目资助的资源，为面临的常见问题实现增值？

● 在每个常见问题的预算范围内，我们能否将资源从价值较低的干预措施转移到价值较高的？

- *Of the activities we do, can we reduce the level of one or more to free resources for?*
- *Could we reduce the purchase cost of some drugs or equipment?*

Thus, value can be increased by addressing these questions and acting upon the answers.

Table 9.2 Budget building; key questions about key resources

Key resource	Comment	Key questions	Key financial issues
Patients	Patients are probably the most neglected resource	• What steps are being taken to provide and support self-care? • Do the patients hold their own records? • Can they request follow up consultations or telephone advice as they feel they require it, or are they scheduled into regular clinic appointments?	Probably no finance identified for patients; there should be a budget for patient information;if there is none, one should be created
Carers	Carers are another neglected resource	• How heavy is the burden on carers? • Dose carer exhaustion play any part in demand on services? • Do carers have all the information they need, including information about access in emergency?	No finance usually identified for carers; as for patients, there should be a budget for carer information
Patient organisations	Patient organisations play an invaluable role in networks of care	• How many national patient organsations are there? • How many, if any, local branches are three of these organisations? • What is the potential for stengthening and expending their contribution?	Patient and carer organisations can be helped without finance, e.g.by the office of rooms for meetings,but small grants give a very good return on investment in patient organisations
General practice	There is a high degree of variation in the clinical practice of general praci-tioners	• What proportion of general practitioners' time is spent on this condition? • What resources do general practitioners feel they lack? • Are there particular general practitioners with special skills or interests who want to do more? • Could general practice trainees be more involved with the service?	The only way to estimate the finanical cost of general practice time is to take the percentage of consulations on the condition and use this to calculate the financial cost of general practice input; this estimate is probably not worth the effort required

- 在我们所进行的各项活动中，是否可以降低一项或多项活动的级别以节约资源？
- 我们能否降低某些药品或设备的采购成本？

因此，通过解决上述问题并将答案付诸行动，就能实现增值。

表9.2 预算编制：与重要资源有关的关键问题

重要资源	解释	关键问题	关键的财务问题
患者	患者是最可能被忽视的资源	<ul><li>正在采取哪些措施支持自我保健？</li><li>患者是否持有自己的健康档案？</li><li>如果患者需要，是否可以请求随诊或电话咨询，或安排到常规的预约门诊？</li></ul>	可能没有固定为患者所用的经费；应该编制患者信息的预算；如果没有，则应该编制此类预算
医疗照护人员	医疗照护人员是另外一类被忽视的资源	<ul><li>照护人员的负担有多重？</li><li>照护人员的过度疲劳会对医疗需求有影响吗？</li><li>照护人员有他们所需要的全部信息吗？包括急诊的就诊信息？</li></ul>	通常没有针对照护人员的经费；如同患者一样，应该编制与卫生保健人员信息相关的预算
患者组织	患者组织在照护网络中发挥着不可估量的作用	<ul><li>国家级的患者组织有多少？</li><li>如果有国家级的患者组织，这些组织在地方上有多少分支机构？</li><li>加强和扩大其作用的潜在好处是什么？</li></ul>	患者和照护人员组织可以得到除经费之外的帮助，如提供会议室。如对患者组织提供小额经费，必定能得到很好的投资回报
全科医生	全科医生的临床实践有着很大程度的差异	<ul><li>在这种情况下，全科医生花费时间占多大比例？</li><li>全科医生认为他们缺少什么资源？</li><li>那些具有专长或对某些方向感兴趣的全科医生想做更多工作吗？</li><li>接受全科培训的人员可以更多地参与这项服务吗？</li></ul>	现有条件下，用就诊时间所占比例这一指标是估算全科医师时间成本的唯一方法，以此还可用于计算全科诊疗投入的财务成本；然而为此类估算投入如此多的精力可能不足为法

续表

Key resource	Comment	Key questions	Key financial issues
Community services	Community services may be based in a community services organisation or works as outreach services from a hospital	● What is the involvement of: -health visitors; -home nurses; -occupational therapists; -physiotherapists; -podiatrists. ● What constraints do these staff face in delivering high value care? ● Who are the leaders within these professional group?	Good data on number of visits and work done,but financial cost may have to be estimated by using the perccentage of work done on the condition in relation to the total budget of community services
Social care	Social care is a key resource even though it may be supported from another financial stream	● How much resource does social care invest in people with this condition? ● What constrations impair social services' ability to be as helpful as the health service thinks they could be? ● In what way could healthcare recources be used to reduce pressure on social care budgets?	Usually very well costed by the local authority
Private care	Private care has more relevance for some health services than others; impacts on health service resources can be both positive and negative	● What private sector resources are used by people with this condition? ● Is the impact on publicly funded services negative or positive? ● How could a clearer understanding between sectors improve the value derived from public resources?	The cost per case,or at least the price charged,is usually public knowledge,the number of cases is not
Pharmacists	The knowledge and skills of pharmacists are probably the most under-used in the healthcare workforce	● How much hospital or specialist pharmacist time is committed to the programme? ● Is there a pharmacist with a special interest or responsibility? ● Could the specialist pharmacist make an even more valuable contribution? ● How many community pharmacists are involved with patients? ● Could their contribution be more valuable with additional training or specialisation?	It is usually simple to cost whole-time equivalents using pharmacists' salaries

续表

重要资源	解释	关键问题	关键的财务问题
社区服务	社区服务可以来自社区医疗机构或来自医院的外展服务	● 涉及的方面： －保健访视员 －家庭护士 －职业治疗师 －理疗师 －足病治疗师 ● 这些工作人员在提供高价值照护服务时会遇到哪些限制？ ● 这些专业团体中的领导者是谁？	尽管已经有了关于访视次数和已完成工作的高质量数据，但是财务成本可能还需要通过与社区服务总预算相关工作和完成的百分比来估算
社会关怀	即使社会关怀的资金支持可能来源于其他渠道，它仍然是一项重要的资源	● 社会关怀为患病人群投入了多少资源？ ● 哪些制约因素削弱了本应和医疗机构发挥相同作用的社会服务机构的能力？ ● 医疗卫生资源可以采用哪种方式来减轻社会关怀的预算压力？	地方政府通常会花很多钱
私人医疗	私人医疗与某些医疗服务的关系更紧密：对医疗服务资源的影响可能是积极的，也可能是消极的	● 此种情况的人群都可以使用哪些私人部门的资源？ ● 公共资助医疗服务产生的是消极影响还是积极影响？ ● 如何通过各部门之间的充分理解来提高公共资源的价值？	通常每个病例的费用或至少定价是众所周知的，但病例数量并不清楚
药剂师	药剂师的知识和技能可能是医疗卫生人员中发挥作用最不充分的	● 医院药剂师或专科药剂师为项目投入了多少时间？ ● 是否有药剂师有特殊兴趣或特定责任？ ● 专科药剂师能做出更有价值的贡献吗？ ● 有多少社区的药剂师是为患者服务的？ ● 额外培训或专业课程是否会使他们的付出更有价值？	用药剂师的工资来衡量其全职工作成本通常是比较容易的

续表

Key resource	Comment	Key questions	Key financial issues
Medication	Medication is often the fastest growing cost	● How many people receive drug treatment? ● How much variation is there in prescribing? ● Where are generic options available and what proportion of prescriptions are generic?	Usually well documented
Specialist clinic	The term "outpatients" is an outdated 19th century term	● How many clinics sessions are there in the year? ● Are all the sessions managed by consultants? ● Assuming a 100% attendance rate,how many consulations can take place in these sessions? ● Are telephone or email consultations and available?	Much more difficult to find down; clinics may not be charged to each specialist service
Hospital beds	Even though hospital beds are not owned by the relevant specialty,an estimate of bed days should be included in the inventory	● What is the average duration of stay? ● How many admissions take place in the course of the year? ● How many bed days are used in the year? ● What proportion of hospital admissions were day case?	Difficult to cost but the finance department are usually able to provide an estimate
Theatre resources	Theatre resources are not applicable to every speciality,they are often difficult to calculate because the relevant operations may be done as part of a long list with other operations	● How many operations were done in the last year? ● What was the cost of equipment used in the operations?	The theatre manager can often provide good costings for a theatre session
Imaging	For some disease,the demand for imaging is growing at a faster rate than that for drugs	● Number of MRIs and rate of increase since previous year ● Number of CTs and rate of increase since previous year ● Number of other images and increase since previous year ● Is there any scope for increasing interventional techniques to reduce the use of other resources?	Some imaging departments have good costings

续表

重要资源	解释	关键问题	关键的财务问题
治疗药物	治疗药物往往是增长最快的成本	● 有多少人接受药物治疗？ ● 处方有多大差别？ ● 有多少种仿制药的选择，在所有处方中有多大比例是仿制药？	通常有完整的记录
专科诊所	"门诊患者"是一个过时的19世纪术语	● 一年有多少次会诊？ ● 所有的会诊都由高年资医师负责吗？ ● 假设会诊的参与率为100%，在这些会诊中有多少次能够进行专业咨询讨论？ ● 患者可以用电话或电子邮件方式咨询和联系医生吗？	很难找到相关数据；诊所可能并不向每项专科服务收费
医院床位	尽管病床不归相关专科所有，但财产清单中应包括床位使用天数估算	● 平均住院时间是多少？ ● 一年中办理住院次数有多少？ ● 一年内有多少床日数？ ● 日间病例占住院人数的比例是多少？	虽然很难计算成本，但财务部门通常还是能够估算
手术室资源	手术室资源并不适用于每个专科；有些手术可能需要与其他手术联合完成。通常很难计算	● 去年做了多少台手术？ ● 在手术中使用设备的费用是多少？	手术室管理者通常应提供合理的手术室成本核算
影像学检查	某些疾病对影像学检查需求的增长速度快于对药物的需求	● 磁共振成像检查的数量以及与往年相比的增长率 ● CT检查的数量以及与往年相比的增长率 ● 其他影像学检查的数量以及与往年相比的增长率 ● 是否存在以增加技术干预措施来减少其他资源的使用？	有些影像部门有合理的成本核算

续表

Key resource	Comment	Key questions	Key financial issues
Laboratory services	More than one estimate may need to be prepared for different types of service, e.g. biochemistry and haematology, depending on the condition	● What are the tests most commonly ordered? ● It is possible to classify the tests as used for either diagnostic or monitoring purposes? ● What is the rate of increase in the five most commonly requested tests	The cost per test may be available but remember to cost the work gengrated by false positive test results
Specialist personnel	Specilalist personnels are the most valuable and expensive resource	● How many whole-time equivalents of: -nursing staff? -medical staff? -physiotherapists? -occupational therapists? -scientists? -managerial staff? -staff in trainning?	The cost can be estimated from the salaries of specialist staff
Real estate	Real estate comprises such items as wards, clinics, and offices, at present, realestate is rarely charged to clinical terms. but this will change	● How much space is occupied by the service as sole occupied? ● How much space do we share with other services? ● Of the space we occupy alone,what proportion of it is not occupied for more than half the time?	Difficult to estimate but can be done by using the proportion of the whole hospital budget that the service represents and then calculating the proportion of the capital value
Information Technology(IT)	Although IT is a consumer of resources, it is also a potential saver of resources	●Does the service have any contracts for IT? ● What proportion of the total IT budget is the service responsible for?	The posibility of costing IT depends on the balance of stand-alone IT to the share of general hospital IT
Management and administration	It is essential to maximise productivity in management and administration, but what is the right level of investment?	●Number of whole-time equivalent administrative and management staff ●National share of central mangement costs, e,g, human resource departments ●Number of whole-time equivalent of professional staff with explicit mangement duties	Staff wholly employed in the service can be calculated; general overheads can be estimated as 50% of clinical staff salaries

续表

重要资源	解释	关键问题	关键的财务问题
实验室检查	根据不同的疾病，可能需要对不同类型的实验室检查（如生物化学和血液学检查）进行多次评估	● 最常见的检查是什么？ ● 可以将检查分为用于诊断目的或者用于监测目的的两大类吗？ ● 五种最常见检测项目的增长率是多少？	每次检测的成本是可以核算的，但也须包括假阳性检测结果的成本
专科医生	专科医生是最宝贵和最昂贵的资源	● 相当于多少个以下人员全职工作时间： －护理人员 －医学专家 －物理治疗师 －职业治疗师 －实验室专家 －管理人员 －接受培训的人员	人员的成本可用专科医生的工资来进行估算
不动产	不动产包括病房、诊所和办公室等；目前，不动产的费用很少由临床团队承担，但这种情况可能会改变	● 有多少空间是完全被使用者单独占用了？ ● 与其他服务共享的空间有多少？ ● 在独占的空间中，使用时间不超过一半的比例是多少？	尽管难以估算不动产的成本，但可以通过某项服务在整个医院预算中所占的比例来进行估算，然后再计算实际固定资本价值所占的比例
信息技术	虽然信息技术是资源的消耗者，但也可以是资源的潜在节约者	● 服务项目与信息技术方面有合同吗？ ● 在总的信息技术预算中，该服务所占的比例是多少？	是否能对信息技术成本进行核算，取决于独立的信息技术与医院综合信息技术共享的程度
管理与行政	最大限度地提高管理和行政的运行效率至关重要，但是合理的投资	● 全职行政和管理人员数 ● 中央管理成本中的名义成本份额，例如人力资源部门 ● 具有明确管理职责的全职专业人员数	全部受雇于该服务的工作人员的成本是可以核算的；日常管理费可用临床工作者工资的50%进行估算

■ Questions for reflection or for use in teaching or network building

If using these questions in network building or teaching, put one of the questions to the group and ask them to work in pairs to reflect on the question for three minutes; try to get people who do not know one another to work together. When taking feedback, let each pair make only one point. In the interests of equity, start with the pair on the left-hand side of the room for responses to the first question, then go to the pair on the right-hand side of the room for responses to the second question.

- How would you organise your first meeting on population-based planning?
- How should common symptoms such as breathlessness be dealt with in a programme budgeting system that assumes every patient has a diagnosis?
- If you were a commissioner faced by a demand for more resources for cataract surgery, how could you relate this bid to other uses, within an eye service, to which the same amount of resources could be put?

References

(1) Seddon, J. (2003) Freedom from Command and Control. Vanguard Education Ltd.

(2) Gardner, H.K. (2012) Performance Pressure as a Double Edged Sword. Administrative Science Quarterly, 57: 1-46.

■ 互动思考题

如果在工作网络建设或教学中使用以下问题，可以将其中一个问题交给小组，让他们两人一组，思考3分钟，并尽量让彼此不认识的人一起工作。要求每组只能提出一个观点作为反馈。为了公平起见，让房间左侧的一组开始回答第1个问题，然后让房间右侧的一组开始回答第2个问题。

- 你将如何组织第一次以人群为基础的财务预算会议？

- 在假定每个患者都有一种疾病的项目预算系统中，应该如何处理像呼吸困难这样的常见症状？

- 若你是一名专员，当白内障手术有更多的资源需求时，你如何将这一需求与需要同等资源但用于其他眼科服务联合起来一并进行考虑呢？

———————————————————————————— 参 考 文 献 ——

（3）Mooney, G.H., Russell, E.M., Weir, R.D.（1980）Choices for Health Care. The Macmillan Press Ltd（pp.10-11）.

Chapter 10
MANAGING KNOWLEDGE

第十章
知识管理

This chapter will:

- Emphasise the benefits of managing knowledge as carefully as one manages money;
- Provide a classificaton of knowledge;
- Describe what can be done without spending more money to manage knowledge better.

By the end of this chapter, you will have developed an understanding of:

- The difference between tacit and explicit knowledge;
- The role and responsibilities of the Chief Knowledge Officer;
- How to realise the potential of librarians;
- How knowledge from experience can be harnessed.

Toyota is a knowledge business.

— President，*Toyota Motor Corporation*

Toyota plans to introduce two electric vehicles in the United States and six hybrid cars worldwide by the end of 2012.

— International Herald Tribune 15.9.2010

■ Healthcare is a knowledge business

It is clear that healthcare is in the business of improving health, just as Toyota is in the business of producing cars, but few people would realise that Toyota's second dimension was in the business of knowledge.

Some people think of healthcare as in the business of real estate — building more hospitals — and some think of it as in the business of technology, such as scanners, drugs and sterilising equipment. However, healthcare is a perfect example of a knowledge business. Although chief executives of hospitals must manage the real estate, they employ 'knowledge' workers, that is, people who add value because they know more about a particular topic than anyone else in the population. It is knowledge that creates the technology, and knowledge that determines when it should be used for best value.

In most health services, however, knowledge is managed much less carefully

本章涉及内容：

- 强调管理知识的受益能够像仔细地管理钱财一样获益；

- 提供一种知识分类方式；

- 阐述在不用花费更多钱财的前提下，我们如何将知识管理得更好。

在本章末，读者将会深入理解：

- 隐性知识和显性知识的区别；

- 首席知识管理官的角色及职责；

- 如何让图书管理员发挥其潜能；

- 如何从经验中获取知识。

丰田是一家知识型企业。

——丰田汽车公司总裁

丰田计划2012年底在美国发布两款电动车，全世界范围内发布六种混合动力车。

——《国际先驱论坛报》2010年9月15日

■ 医疗保健是知识型行业

很明显，医疗卫生保健是一个改善健康的行业，这就好像丰田是从事生产汽车的行业一样。但是，几乎没有人能认识到，丰田还是一家知识型企业。

尽管有人认为医疗卫生行业是不动产行业，例如建更多的医院；也有人将其视为技术型行业，如使用扫描仪、药物和消毒设备。但从实际上来讲，医疗卫生领域是知识型行业的完美范例。虽然首席执行官必须管理医院，但他们聘用的是"知识型"工作者，是比其他人更了解特定知识而为医院带来价值的人。知识创造了技术，知识决定了技术的最佳使用时机。

在大多数医疗照护中，管理知识的仔细程度远逊于管理资金或建筑物。

than money or buildings. It is relatively easy to discover the name of every estates manager in the NHS, but not the name of every knowledge manager. Indeed, in many NHS organisations, no-one has this responsibility.

■ Knowledge management responsibilities in population medicine

As knowledge is critically important in achieving good outcomes for patients and in maximising value from clinical services, clinicians with managerial responsibilities (whole-or part-time) should include a responsibility for managing knowledge in their brief, and assume this responsibility if it has not been given to them. Furthermore, as knowledge is shared and exchanged in populations, such clinicians should take responsibility for the management of knowledge for the whole population, not just for those patients in contact with the service.

The management of knowledge for the population is one of the key responsibilities and new skills of population medicine, partly because any service is in competition with other providers. The traditional responsibility towards knowledge management is that all professionals who work within the specialist service should be up to date with best current evidence. This type of responsibility, however, is focussed on self-improvement for a limited number of individuals and could have potentially negative consequences for the care of the population served. In this situation, it is not clear who has overall responsibility for meeting the information needs of the wider community of clinicians serving the population in need (see Display 10.1). Part of the reason for a lack of clarity about who is responsible for managing knowledge for the population is that certain specific responsibilities for information provision may rest with different healthcare professionals.

Display 10.1 A population-based clinical practice simulation

Scenario: You are a clinician with responsibility for orthopaedic and rheumatology services for a population of 500,000 people who is responsible for ensuring that:

- a new general practitioner in the population served knows the referral criteria for back pain?
- patients are assured that the service provided in their locality serves them better than the service in the neighbouring locality?
- the hip re-operation rate in your locality is within an acceptable range?
- older people in the population know about fragility fractures and how they can be prevented?
- pharmacists and general practitioners know the best-value drug treatment for rheumatoid arthritis?
- people who make decisions about licensing alcohol understand what they can do to prevent trauma?
- patients considering knee replacement understand the probability and nature of the risks of the operation as well as they understand the benefits?
- when surgeons retire, the key lessons they have learnt are captured and passed on?

在NHS体系内，找到每个不动产管理者的姓名相对容易，但是找到每个知识
管理者的姓名就没那么容易了。实际上，在NHS体系内的医疗卫生组织中，
没有人承担这项职责。

■ 群医学中知识管理的职责

由于知识在临床诊疗中为患者带来良好结果和最大价值极为重要，承担
着管理职责的临床医生（无论全职或兼职）即使没有被赋予知识管理的职责，
也应在其工作简报中包括这项任务。此外，知识是在人群中交流共享的，上
述临床医生不仅应为求医患者进行知识管理，还应为有需求的全体人群负责。

为人群管理知识是群医学的一项关键职责和全新技能，部分原因是任何
服务都在与其他提供者竞争。知识管理的传统职责是，在专科工作的所有专
业人员都应该不停地更新最新的证据。但是，由于担负知识管理职责的人仅
聚焦于少数人的自我完善，这可能会给接受医疗的人群带来潜在不良后果。
在这种情况下，现在还不清楚到底应该由谁来满足广大临床医生团体的信息
需求（场景10.1）。此事尚不明晰的部分原因是：提供信息的特定职责可能分
属于不同的医疗卫生人员。

场景10.1 以人群为基础的临床实践模拟

情况：您是一名临床医生，负责为50万人提供骨科疾病和风湿病的服务。你要为下列问题负责：
● 新全科医生知道他所服务的人群有关背痛的转诊标准吗？
● 与周边地区相比，患者是否知道当地为他们提供了更好的医疗吗？
● 所在地区的髋关节再手术率是否在可接受的范围内？
● 人群中的老年人了解脆性骨折以及如何预防吗？
● 药剂师和全科医生了解类风湿关节炎最佳药物治疗措施吗？
● 批准酒精类销售许可证的决策者知道采取什么措施来预防创伤吗？
● 考虑做膝关节置换的患者了解手术风险、性质以及好处吗？
● 外科医生在退休时，他们学到的主要经验教训会被保留并传承下去吗？

The roles and responsibilities of three types of clinician in relation to knowledge provision are shown in Table 10.1, however, each role needs to be developed and the coordination among them improved.

Table 10.1 Roles and responsilbilities for knowledge provision for three groups of healthcare professionals

Healthcare professional and their responsibility to knowledge provision	Action required
General practitioners have a dear responsibility to ensure that: ● they have access to best current knowledge; ● the patients who attend for consultations receive the knowledge they need.	In a health centre at which there is a team of general practitioners and other clinicians, one clinician should take lead responsibility and adopt the role of Chief Knowledge Officer.
Specialist clinicians working in hospitals or mental health services have an important part to play in ensuring that all patients directly supported by the service receive information about their condition, and the probability of the benefit and the harm relating to the different treatment options for their condition.	Clinicians who are medical managers of a service should consider the knowledge needs of: ● staff in the specialist service; ● general practitioners, particularly those new to the locality; ● pharmacists in private community pharmacies; ● physiotherapists in the community service and private practice; ● patients who reach the service.
Directors of public health have a responsibility for delivering public health services to a defined population. Just as it is a public health responsibility to ensure that the population has clean water so should it be a responsibility for the pulbic health service to ensure clear knowledge? (1)	Directors of public health must ensure that everyone in the local population (induding people who do not have a general practitioner) receives the knowledge they need, particularly knowledge relating to how to stay healthy and prevent disease.

■ Knowledge as a driver for better value healthcare

Manual Castells has described three eras of industrial revolution(2), an analysis that can be applied to the evolution of healthcare.

- *The first industrial revolution was driven by empirical commonsense James Watt did not understand the physics of steam but drew conclusions from the boiling of his mother's kettle; in the first healthcare revolution, John Snow did not know that the causative agent of cholera was Vibrio cholerae, but he did work out that the cases of cholera were linked to water from the Broad Street pump.*

表10.1列出了3类临床医生在提供知识方面的角色和职责。但是，各角色仍需开发，并且需要增进彼此之间的协调。

表10.1 3组医疗卫生专业人员在提供知识方面的角色和职责

医疗卫生专业人员及 知识提供职责	需要采取的行动
全科医生有一项明确的职责，即确保： ● 自己能够获得最好最新的知识； ● 就医患者能获得所需的知识。	在由全科医生和其他临床医生组成的医疗中心，由一名临床医生承担主要责任并担任首席知识官。
在医院或精神卫生医疗机构工作的专科医生有一个重要角色，即确保该服务部门直接照护的所有患者都获得有关自己病情的信息以及不同治疗方案可能带来的损益概率。	医疗机构管理岗的临床医生应考虑以下人员的知识需求： ● 从事专科医疗的员工； ● 全科医生，特别是本地新来的全科医生； ● 社区私人药房的药剂师； ● 在社区服务和私人执业中的物理治疗师； ● 寻求医疗照护的患者。
公共卫生部门主任负责为特定人群提供公共卫生服务。正如确保人群拥有干净清洁的水是公共卫生的一项职责，确保获得清晰明确的知识难道不也应该是公共卫生职责之一吗？[1]	公共卫生部门主任必须确保当地人群中的每个人（包括未与全科医生签约的人）均能够获得所需的知识，尤其是如何保持健康和预防疾病方面的知识。

■ 知识是提高医疗卫生价值的驱动力

曼纽尔·卡斯特描述了3次工业革命时代[2]，这一分析同样适用于医疗卫生领域的演变。

● 第一次工业革命是由经验常识推动的，詹姆斯·瓦特并不明白蒸汽的物理原理，而是从他母亲沸腾的水壶中得出结论；在第一次医疗卫生革命中，约翰·斯诺并不知道霍乱的病因是霍乱弧菌，但他确实发现霍乱病例与宽街水泵的水有关。

- *The second industrial revolution was driven by scientific advances; during the second healthcare revolution over the last 50 years, notable scientific advances are hip replacement and transplantation.*
- *The third industrial revolution is already taking place and is being driven by three forces: knowledge, the Internet and citizens (Figure 10.1); these drivers are also highly relevant to healthcare, and in particular to population medicine.*

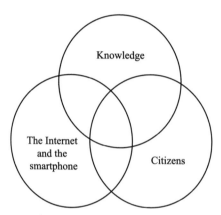

Figure 10.1 Drivers of the Third Healthcare Revolution

It is not common for a clinician to face competition when designing and creating systems and networks for a population but, when trying to ensure that all professionals and patients within a population receive unbiased, clearly presented, up-to-date knowledge, the clinician practising population medicine faces intense competition from the media, particularly the Internet. Key features of the sources of competition to unbiased information about healthcare are shown in Box 10.1.

It is therefore necessary for those who pay for or manage healthcare resources to compete with other sources of knowledge in the knowledge 'marketplace' particularly the Internet.

■ Classifying knowledge

A simple classification of the different types of knowledge is shown in Figure 10.2. Generalisable knowledge can be classified into several categories (see Figure 10.2).

- 第二次工业革命是由科学进步推动的：过去50年的第二次医疗卫生革命中，在髋关节置换和移植方面取得了显著的科学进展。

- 第三次工业革命正在发生，并受到三股力量的驱动：知识、互联网和民众（图10.1）。这些驱动因素也与医疗卫生，特别是群医学，高度相关。

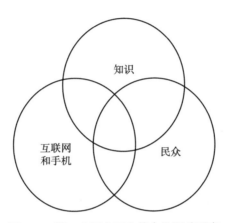

图10.1　第三次医疗卫生革命的驱动因素

在为人群设计和创建相关系统和网络时，临床医生很少遇到竞争。相反，当试图确保人群中所有专业人员和患者获取客观公正、清晰表述、及时更新的知识时，从事群医学的临床医生要面临着来自媒体，尤其是互联网的激烈竞争。对于客观公正的医疗卫生信息，其竞争来源的主要特征如图10.1所示。

因此，对于购买或管理医疗卫生资源的人来说，有必要与知识"市场"中的其他知识来源相竞争，尤其是互联网。

■ 知识分类

图10.2简要描述了不同知识的分类。通识可进一步分为以下几类（图10.2）。

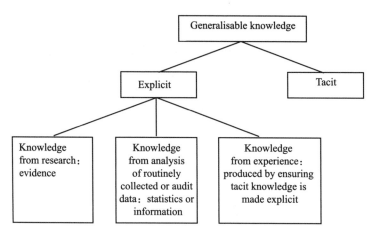

Figure 10.2　Three types of explicit knowledge

■ Managing different types of knowledge

The management of knowledge involves not only its creation but also its use, both of which require good management. In health services, the management of all types of generalisable knowledge needs to be improved.

■ Improving the management of knowledge from experience

Tacit knowledge consists partly of technical skills — the kind of informal, hard-to-pin down skills captured in the term 'knowhow'.

A master craftsman after years of experience develops a wealth of exper-tise'at his finger-tips'. But he is often unable to articulate the scientific or technical principles behind what he knows.

At the same time, tacit knowledge has an important cognitive dimension. It consists of mental models, beliefs, and perspectives so ingrained that we take them for granted, and therefore cannot easily articulate them. (3)

■ Knowledge from the experience of professionals

Of the three types of explicit knowledge, knowledge from experience is the type least well managed. It needs to be created by converting tacit knowledge into explicit forms, for example, by:

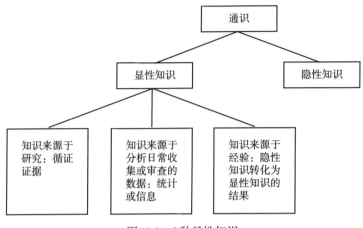

图10.2　3种显性知识

■ 管理不同类型的知识

知识管理不仅包括创造，还包括应用，而两者均需要良好的管理。在医疗卫生中，所有类型的知识管理都需要提高。

■ 改善来源于经验的知识管理

隐性知识包括技术技能——一种非正式的、难以确定的技能，即所谓的"诀窍"。

有多年经验的熟练工匠具有丰富的专业知识，"唯手熟尔"，但通常他无法阐述其背后的科学或技术原理。

同时，隐性知识具有重要的认知维度，它由思维模式、信念和观点组成。这些认知往往根深蒂固，以至于我们将其视为理所当然而无法轻易表达出来[3]。

■ 来自专业人员经验的知识

在3类显性知识中，来自经验的知识是最不好管理的。以下方式可以将隐性知识转化为显性知识：

- *interviewing staff as they leave (exit interviews or knowledge harvesting) to find out what their successor needs to know and how the service could change for the better;*
- *celebrating successes and profiting from failures by ensuring that there is time for reflection and discussion after a project is finished;*
- *building a casebook in which people record the outcomes of projects, successful and unsuccessful, and the lessons learned;*
- *developing partnerships with other services and arranging exchanges so that members of staff can experience different approaches to the same job in different contexts;*
- *using the Map of Medicine and other software for care pathways to make tacit knowledge explicit in a graphic medium, which is much more accessible for the majority of people.*

In addition to these formal techniques of converting tacit to explicit knowledge, learning can be garnered during informal situations. The clinician leading a service needs to create a culture in which discussing the service in a social setting is seen as valuable. The cultural change required is one best described as the transformation to a learning organisation.

Peter Senge, who popularized learning organizations in his book The Fifth Discipline, described them as places 'where people continually expand their capacity to create the results they truly desire, where new and expansive patterns of thinking are nurtured, where collective aspiration is set free, and where people are continually learning how to learn together'. In a similar spirit Ikujiro Nonaka characterized knowledge-creating companies as places where 'inventing new knowledge is not a specialized activity. ...it is a way of behaving, indeed a way of being, in which everyone is a knowledge worker. A learning organization is an organization skilled at creating, acquiring and transferring knowledge, and at modifying its behaviour to reflect new knowledge and insights'. (4)

Within healthcare, the concept of the learning organisation has been promoted by the Institute of Medicine (part of the US National Academies of Science), which produces helpful publications on the topic. The Institute has described the 'Learning Healthcare System' as:

- 对离职员工进行访谈（离职采访或知识收集），了解其继任者所需的知识和如何将服务变得更好；
- 庆祝成功，吸取失败教训，确保在项目完成后有时间进行反思和讨论；
- 编写案例集，记录成功和失败的项目结果，以及所获得的经验教训；
- 与其他医疗机构发展伙伴关系并安排交流活动，使工作人员体验到不同背景下相同工作的不同做法；
- 使用医学地图（Map of Medicine®）或临床路径的其他软件，通过图形媒介使隐性知识变得清晰，便于大多数人学习。

除了上述将隐性知识转化为显性知识的正规方式外，也可在非正式情况下获得知识。临床医生作为医疗机构的领导者，需要创造一种文化，在这种文化中，在社会环境下讨论医疗服务被认为有价值的。转变为学习型组织是对这种文化所需变化的最好诠释。

彼得·圣吉在其《第五项修炼》中推广了学习型组织，将此类机构描述为"在这里，人们不断扩展能力以创造自己真正想要的结果；在这里，全新广阔的思维模式被培育；在这里，集体意愿被释放出来；在这里，人们不断学习如何共同学习"。野中郁次郎提出了内核相近的观点，将知识创造型企业描述为"创造新知识不是一项专门的工作……而是一种行为方式，实际上是一种存在方式，每个人都是知识工作者。学习型组织是一个善于创造、获取和传输知识，并善于改变其行为以反映新知识和洞见的组织"。[4]

在医疗卫生领域，医学研究所（美国国家科学院的一部分）推广了学习型组织的概念，该研究所就这一主题发布了有指导意义的出版物，其将"学习型医疗卫生系统"描述如下：

The fundamental notion of the learning healthcare system — continuous improvement in effectiveness, efficiency, safety, and quality — is rooted in principles that medicine shares with engineering. The goal of a learning healthcare system is to deliver the best care every time, and to learn and improve with each care experience. (5)

■ Knowledge from the experience of patients

The importance of harnessing the knowledge of patients, not only for the purposes of learning but also as part of developing an emotional bond with patients, has been emphasised elsewhere in this book (see Chapter 8).

Improving the management of knowledge from evidence. Evidence is generally considered to be information from clinical experience that has met some established test of validity, and the appropriate standard is determined according to the requirements of the intervention and clinical circumstance. (6)

The definition of evidence quoted above highlights the distinction between evidence from research and evidence from experience: evidence from research requires a 'test of validity'. Both types of knowledge, however, are needed in healthcare. Clinicians worldwide have adopted the paradigm of evidence-based decision-making, and in particular evidence-based medicine. Evidence-based medicine (EBM):

...requires the integration of the best research evidence with our clinical expertise and our patient's unique values and circumstances. (7)

This conception of EBM can be represented graphically (see Figure 10.3).

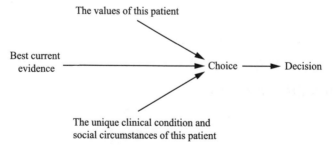

Figure 10.3 The three contributors to informed choice

学习型医疗卫生系统的基本理念——不断提高效果、效率、安全和质量——根植于医学与工程共享的原则。学习型医疗卫生系统的目标是保证每次均能提供最佳照护，并根据每次照护的经验进行学习和改进[5]。

■ 来自患者体验的知识

本书第八章强调了利用患者知识的重要性，这不仅是为了学习的目的，也是与患者建立情感纽带的一部分。

从证据中加强对知识的管理。证据通常来源于满足一些有效性测试的临床经验，而合适的标准是根据干预措施和临床环境的要求确定的。[6]

上述证据的定义突出了研究证据与经验证据的区别——从研究得到的证据需要"有效性测试"。然而，这两种类型的知识都是医疗卫生领域所需要的。世界各地的临床医生采用了循证的决策模式，特别是循证医学的模式。

循证医学（evidence-based medicine，EBM）要求把最佳研究证据、临床专家意见、患者个人独特的价值观和具体情况整合在一起[7]。

循证医学的概念如图所示（图10.3）。

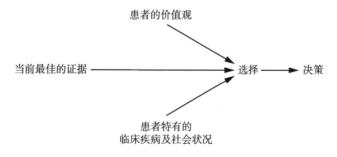

图10.3 影响选择的3个因素

Evidence-based medicine, however, has been supplemented and complemented by evidence-based management to enable clinicians to incorporate the evidence-based paradigm into clinical practice.

...evidence based management [is the] knowledge of how to put [evidence based medicine] into practice...it focuses on the underlying organisational issues that influence how care is delivered. The evidence base comes largely from the social and behavioural sciences, human factors engineering and the fields of health services research. In addition to RCT's [sic] evidence based evidence management uses observational data and methods such as PDCA.（8）

The medical manager needs to take four steps to facilitate and improve evidence-based clinical decision-making（see Box 10.1）.

Box 10.1 Steps to facilitate and improve evidence-based clinical decision-making

1. Support the development of the clinical skills of inexperienced clinicians to enable them to relate the evidence from research to the unique clinical condition and social circumstances of the patient — 'personalised medicine', articulated by Peter Rothwell as a question 'How can I judge whether the probability of benefit from treatment in my current patient is likely to differ substantially from the average probability of benefit reported in the relevant trial or systematic review?'（9）. Do not assume that clinicians are better at understanding risk than patients because statistical illiteracy — 'the inability of many physicians, patients, journalists and politicians alike to understand what health statistics mean'（10）is common

2. Provide patients and clinicians with clear up-to-date information

3. Provide patients and clinicians with decision aids to support decision-making when the patient's values are of vital importance, and in particular if consultation time is limited

4. Ensure that best current evidence is delivered when and where it is needed; knowledge delivery should be 'just-in-time', especially as there is an increasing number of staff working part-time. Ways to deliver evidence/knowledge just in time include:（i）embedding it in documents such as laboratory request forms, laboratory reports, or letters to clinical colleagues and patients;（ii）using what are called 'forcing functions' in the safety literature — *'...reminders or constraints that suggest or require a certain response from the person using the machine'*（11） — for example, introducing into a process an evidence-based check that a clinician must complete before proceeding

5. Ensure that the evidence base used by each service is regularly updated; an annual update is usually sufficient, except in the case of safety alerts, which should be incorporated and communicated immediately

在经历循证管理的补充完善后，循证医学使临床医生能够在临床实践中纳入循证行医范式。

……循证管理（是）一类如何将（循证医学）付诸实践的知识……它聚焦于潜在组织问题，而这些问题影响了医疗卫生供给。其证据基础主要来自社会和行为科学、人因（人为因素）工程学以及医疗卫生照护研究领域。除了随机对照试验方法外，循证管理也采用可观察的数据和其他方法，如PDCA。[8]

医疗卫生管理者需要采取4个步骤以促进和改进循证临床决策过程（专栏10.1）。

专栏10.1　促进与优化循证临床决策的步骤

1. 提升经验不足的临床医生的临床技能，使他们能够将研究证据与患者独特的临床指征和社会状况联系起来——即彼得·罗斯韦尔所描述的"个性化医学"，他提出"我如何判断当前患者从治疗中受益的概率是否与相关试验或系统综述中的平均受益概率有很大差异？"。[9]不要以为临床医生就比患者更加理解风险，因为"统计文盲"——"许多医生、患者、记者和政治家都无法理解健康统计数据的含义"[10]是常见的。

2. 为患者和临床医生提供清晰、即时的信息。

3. 在患者的看法至关重要时，特别是咨询时间有限的情况下，为患者和临床医生提供决策辅助，以支持临床决策。

4. 确保能在任何时间和地点提供当前最佳证据。提供知识应该是"及时的"，特别是在越来越多的工作人员从事兼职工作的情况下。及时提供证据或知识的方式包括：①将其写入实验室须知表格、实验室报告或告知临床同事及患者的信件中；②使用安全性相关文献中提及的"强制函数——"……建议或要求机器使用者提供某些反馈的提醒或约束机制[11]——例如，引入循证检查是临床医生在进行决策前必须完成的环节。

5. 确保各医疗卫生行为使用的基础证据能够定期更新：通常情况下，每年一次的更新频率是适宜的，但是安全警报除外，安全警报应该即时更新并传达。

■ Improving the management of knowledge from data

Hitherto, the information used by managers has been restricted to finance and activity data. In the 21st century, the priority will be to manage services using information about quality and outcome.

Information on quality can be collected through audits undertaken in the institution in which the medical manager works. To obtain information on outcomes, which is essential for the assessment of value, data inputs from the whole system of care are required. For instance, to gain information about the outcome of hip replacement, data are required about:

- *the pre-operative health status of the individual*;
- *the individual's health status three months after the hip has been replaced, long after the patient has left hospital.*

Thus, obtaining information about outcomes, including clinical measures and patient-reported outcome measures, requires the cooperation of the entire network of services providing care for the population, and of individual patients seen by the service.

The debate about the relative importance of process and outcome measures has attracted much attention. There is now a consensus that, although both are necessary, in future people who manage healthcare will be held to account not only for the quality and safety of the care they provide to patients but also for the value derived from the resources. There are two ways in which to estimate value:

1. by relating outcome to expenditure;

2. by comparing services, and plotting the position of each service on the value map shown in Figure 10.4.

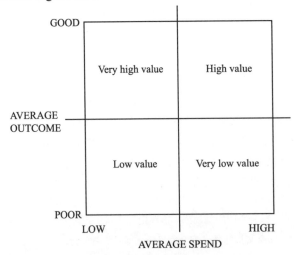

Figure 10.4 The value matrix

■ 从数据中改进知识管理

迄今为止,管理者使用的信息仅局限于财务和活动数据。在21世纪,首要任务将是使用有关质量和结局的信息来管理医疗服务。

关于质量的信息可通过对医疗管理者所工作的机构进行评估来收集。为了获取对价值评估至关重要的结果信息,需要输入来自整个医疗系统的数据。例如,为了获得髋关节置换手术结局的信息,则需要以下数据:

● 患者术前健康状况;

● 髋关节置换3个月后、出院很久后的健康状况。

因此,要获得包括临床评估和患者报告的结局评估在内的有关结局的信息,就需要为人群提供医疗照护的整个网络体系以及接受医疗的个体患者之间的合作。

关于过程和结局评估孰轻孰重的争论由来已久。虽然两者都实属必要,但现已达成共识:未来,医疗卫生管理者不仅为患者的医疗照护质量和安全性负责,还要为从资源中获取的价值负责。可以通过以下两种方式评估价值:

1.将结局和支出挂钩。

2.比较各种医疗服务,在价值图上绘制每种医疗卫生服务的位置(图10.4)。

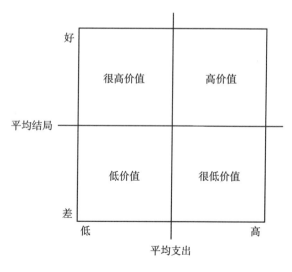

图10.4 价值矩阵

It is vital to assess effectiveness in relation to expenditure; indeed, it could be considered negligent not to do so. Even quality improvement, the target of the last decade, needs to be assessed in relation to the cost of achieving any change in the level of performance. Bob Brook, one of the creators of the quality movement, signalled the end of the quality improvement era in 2010 when he published an article subtitled 'Long Live Increasing Value' (12). The measurement of quality is the means by which institutions can be held to account. The assessment of value, however, requires knowledge to be related to populations and not to institutions.

■ Improving the management of population-based and not just institution-based knowledge

The principle of population accountability was first developed by Mark Friedman (13). Friedman identified the overlap of, but difference between, outcomes for 'populations' and outcomes for 'customers and communities'. Although Friedman's focus is education, his analysis is relevant to healthcare, especially the relationship between population and performance accountability, which can be directly transferred into a healthcare setting (see Table 10.2)

In an era of resource constraint, it is important to create what has been called 'public value for the population' (14) in addition to providing value for individual patients using the service. The creation of value is critical in a context of increasing demands for transparency from both Government and civil society. The objective of transparency as defined by Manson and O'Neill is to improve levels of trust:

Transparency or openness is supplied to improve trustworthiness by exposing misleading claims or failing performance and by creating incentives for institutions and office-holders to be trustworthy, thereby discouraging attempts to play upon others' gullibility in order to gain an unearned reputation for trustworthiness. An expectation of disclosure creates clear incentives for proper behaviour. But by itself transparency does not provide the evidence that is needed to support the intelligent placing and refusal of trust. (15)

Leadership needs to be provided by the Chief Knowledge Officer.

评估与支出相关的效果是很重要的；实际上，不做评估可视为工作的疏漏。即使改善质量（过去十年的工作目标）也需要评估取得成效所带来的成本。质量运动的创建者之一鲍勃·布鲁克在2010年发表了一篇《增加价值万岁》的文章，标志着改善质量时代的结束[12]。评估质量是使医疗机构承担责任的手段，然而评估价值则需要与人群而非医疗机构相关的知识。

■ 改善以人群为基础而不仅是以机构为基础的知识管理

马克·弗里德曼最早提出了人群责任制的原理[13]。弗里德曼确定了"人群"的结果与"客户和社区"的结果之间彼此重叠，但有所差异。尽管弗里德曼的重点是在教育方面，但他的分析与医疗卫生也相关，尤其是可以直接把人群与绩效责任之间的关系转移到医疗卫生领域中（表10.2）。

在资源受限的年代，除了为就诊的个体患者提供价值外，重要的是要创造所谓的"人群公共价值"[14]。在政府和社会对透明度要求越来越高的背景下，创造价值至关重要。如曼森和奥尼尔所界定的，透明的目的是提高信任度：

为提高其可信度，采用透明或公开的方式揭露误导性宣传或失败的业绩，以及通过为公共机构及公职人员创造激励机制，从而阻止那些企图利用他人的轻信而不劳而获得到"值得信赖"声誉的机构或人员。预期此类的披露会创造一种明确的激励机制以端正其行为。但就其本身而言，透明度并不能提供所需要的证据以支持人们是否会明智地选择或拒绝信任[15]。

首席知识官需要具有领导力。

Table 10.2 The relationship between population and performance accountability

The seven population accountability questions	*The seven performance accountability questions*
● What are the quality of life conditions we want for our children, adults and families who live in our community? ● What would those conditions look like if we could see them? ● How can we measure those conditions? ● How are we doing on the most important of these measures? ● Who are the partners that have a role to play in doing better? ● What works to do better, including no-cost and low-cost ideas? ● What do we propose to do?	● Who are our customers? ● How can we measure if our customers are better off? ● How can we measure if we are delivering services well? ● How are we doing on the most important of these measures? ● Who are the partners that have a role to play in doing better? ● What works to do better, including no-cost and low-cost ideas? ● What do we propose to do?

■ The need for a Chief Knowledge Officer

As knowledge is an important resource in any organisation, the management of knowledge requires leadership, and a senior member of staff should be given overall responsibility for managing it. This responsibility can be encapsulated within the role of a Chief Knowledge Officer (16), which was first developed by the private sector in the United States. It is important to emphasise that the Chief Knowledge Officer is a leadership role, not a job. A member of the Senior Management Team, preferably a person directly accountable to the Chief Executive, should be given the responsibility for ensuring that knowledge created and used by an organisation is well managed. If knowledge in the organisation is not well managed, the Chief Knowledge Officer should be given a budget and the authority to mobilise resources to rectify the situation.

In a healthcare setting, the Medical Director is usually the person best qualified to be given the role and responsibility of Chief Knowledge Officer. In turn, the Chief Knowledge Officer can ask each clinical director to take on the corresponding role and responsibility for the relevant directorates. Although it is possible to combine the role and responsibility of a Chief Knowledge Officer with those of a Chief Information Officer, the latter post is usually restricted to the management of data and the production of financial and activity information for management. The typical responsibilities of a Chief Knowledge Officer in a healthcare setting are shown in Box 10.2.

表10.2　人群与绩效责任制的关系

7个人群责任制的问题	7个绩效责任制的问题
● 我们希望为住在社区中的儿童、成人以及家庭提供什么质量的生活条件？	● 我们的客户是谁？
● 如果我们能看到这些条件时，它们是什么样呢？	● 对那些客户境况较好，我们该如何评估我们的客户是否获益更多？
● 我们如何评估这些条件？	● 我们该如何评估我们是否能更好地提供照护？
● 我们对评估工作中最重要的方面做得如何？	● 我们在评估工作中最重要的方面做得如何？
● 谁是我们改善工作的伙伴？	● 当我们想把工作做得更好时，谁是我们的合作伙伴？
● 哪些方法可以做得更好？包括无成本和低成本方法。	● 哪些方法可以做得更好？包括无成本和低成本的方法。
● 我们应该做什么？	● 我们应该做什么？

■ 对首席知识官的需求

由于知识在任何组织中都是一种重要的资源，知识的管理需要领导才能，而一名高级职员应被赋予全面管理知识的职责。首席知识官的角色中包括这类职责[16]。这个职位最初由美国私营部门设置。值得强调的是，首席知识官是一种领导角色，而非一项工作。高级管理团队的一名成员，最好是直接向首席执行官负责的人，应负责确保组织所创造和使用的知识得到妥善管理。如果组织中的知识管理不善，管理团队应给首席知识官预算和授权来调用资源纠正这种情况。

在医疗机构中，医务主任通常是最有资格担任首席知识官角色和职责的人。反之，首席知识官可以要求每位临床主任在其所管辖的部门中承担相应的角色和责任。尽管可将首席知识官和首席信息官的角色和责任结合起来，但后者岗位通常仅限于数据、财务成果和活动信息的管理。专栏10.2列出了首席知识官在医疗机构中的典型职责。

Box 10.2 Responsibilities of a Chief Knowledge Officer in a healthcare setting

- Capturing the tacit knowledge within and about the service and making sure it is used
- Identifying and procuring the sources of evidence that the service requires
- Ensuring that all information for patients is unbiased and clear
- Developing the annual reports for clinical systems and services
- Identifying the wider community of professionals caring for the population served by the service and ensuring their knowledge needs are ascertained and met
- Ensuring the Board and Senior Management Team base their decisions on best current evidence

The aim of a Chief Knowledge Officer is to get knowledge into action, an activity increasingly characterised as knowledge translation, defined by the Canadian Institute of Health Research as 'a dynamic and iterative process that includes synthesis, dissemination, exchange and ethically sound application of knowledge'. (17) In an era when financial resources are constrained, the infinite resource that is knowledge can increase value for the population and for individual patients. (18)

The British Standards Institution (BSI) has produced a Guide to Good Practice in Knowledge Management (19), in which are identified the qualities that a Chief Knowledge Officer might need (see Box 10.3).

Box 10.3 Qualities for a Chief Knowledge Officer

- A 'frontline' background
- The ability to command the respect of senior management
- A deep understanding of the organisation's business and culture
- A high level of technological literacy
- A tolerance of ambiguity and the ability to work with minimal structure

■ Directors of public health as Chief Knowledge Officers for health knowledge

On 28 July 2010, through Resolution 64/292, the United Nations General Assembly recognised the human right to water and sanitation, and acknowledged that clean drinking water and sanitation are essential to the realisation of all human rights (20). Knowledge is like water. Everyone has a need for and a right to clean clear knowledge, in the same way that they have a need for and a right to clean clear water.

专栏10.2　首席知识官在医疗机构中的职责

- 获取医疗服务内部和相关的隐性知识并确保其使用。
- 识别并获得医疗服务所需的证据来源。
- 确保为患者提供的所有信息公正、客观且清晰。
- 编制临床系统和医疗照护的年度报告。
- 确定更为广泛的负责照护人群的专业人员范围，并确保识别和满足他们的知识需求。
- 确保董事会和高级管理团队的决策是建立在现有最佳证据之上的。

首席知识官的目标是将知识付诸行动，这种活动越来越多地从知识转化为特征，加拿大卫生研究院将其定义为：一个动态且迭代的过程，在应用时，应包括知识的综合、传播、交流和合乎伦理的应用。[17]在财政资源受限的时代，知识作为无限资源，可为人群和个体患者增加价值。[18]

英国标准协会（BSI）编写了《知识管理的良好实践指南》，其中确定了首席知识官可能需要的素质（专栏10.3）。

专栏10.3　首席知识官的素质

- 具有"临床一线"背景；
- 有能力得到高层管理人员的尊重；
- 对组织的事业和文化有深刻的了解；
- 高水平的技术素养；
- 能够容忍模棱两可，并有能力与最简结构的团队开展工作。

■ 作为首席知识官的公共卫生主任应具有的医疗卫生知识

2010年7月28日，联合国大会通过第64/292号决议，承认清洁饮用水和卫生设施对于实现人权至关重要[20]。知识就像水，每个人都离不开它，而且有权利得到清晰、明确的知识。正如每个人也需要并有权得到清洁和干净的水。

Ignorance is like cholera, a water-borne disease, it cannot be managed by any one individual; it requires the organised efforts of society. Thus, it is a public health responsibility. The responsibility for ensuring that everyone in the population — professionals, patients and the public — has access to clean clear knowledge could be added to the existing responsibilities of directors of public health. This new responsibility could be discharged through the traditional public health method of needs assessment: by identifying groups whose needs for knowledge are not being adequately met and then through the performance management of Trusts with the main responsibility for delivering knowledge to clinicians and patients who have reached the Trusts' services.

In addition, to ensure that clean clear knowledge is available everywhere, directors of public health could work with:

- *the public library service*;
- *social services*;
- *the third sector of voluntary and community organisations.*

■ Support for the Chief Knowledge Officer: releasing the librarian's potential

It is not possible for the person assigned the role of Chief Knowledge Officer to fulfil all the tasks required without support. The continuing transformation of the library service, with the advent of digital technology and the capacity to deliver documents to any user electronically, opens up the possibility of releasing some of the librarians' time to become knowledge managers for the organisation, with direct accountability to the Chief Knowledge Officer. The librarian is the most valuable resource in the library, and a librarian's skills are too valuable to be confined to that setting. Librarians of the 21st century, however, need to supplement their existing skill set and master new skills to enable them to undertake new tasks (see Box 10.4).

Box 10.4 Tasks for 21st century librarians as knowledge managers

1. Teaching critical appraisal to clinicians and managers
2. Knowledge harvesting
3. Managing the storage, updating and distribution of guidelines
4. Identifying the evidence needs of different departments and developing an evidence service for each
5. Coordinating the patient information service

无知就像霍乱，是一种经"水"传播的疾病。它不能由任何个体管理；而需要社会有组织的努力。因此，这是一项公共卫生责任，确保人群中的每一个人——专业人员、患者和公众——均可以获取清晰、明确的知识，并将这一责任纳入公共卫生主任现有的职责中。可以通过传统的对公共卫生需求进行评估来履行这一新的职责：通过确定那些人还未充分满足其知识需求，解决的办法可以用医疗卫生机构绩效管理的方法，向临床医生和寻求服务的患者们提供知识。

此外，为确保各地均可获得清晰、明确的知识，公共卫生主任可以与下列各机构进行合作：

- 公共图书馆；

- 各种社会服务机构；

- 志愿组织和社区组织等第三方机构。

■ 对首席知识官的支持：发挥图书馆的潜能

被委任首席知识官职责的人不可能在没有支持的情况下完成所有所需的任务。公共图书馆的持续性变革，伴随着数字化技术的出现以及将电子化文件传送给用户的能力，开启了一种节约部分图书管理员的时间以使其成为该组织的知识管理者的可能性，他们可对首席知识官直接负责。图书管理员是图书馆中最有价值的资源，图书管理员的技能太宝贵而不能仅被限制在图书馆中。然而，21世纪的图书管理员需要对他们已有的技能进行完善，并精通新技能以承担新的任务（专栏10.4）。

专栏10.4　21世纪图书管理员作为知识管理者的任务

- 教导临床医生和管理者做批判性评估；
- 知识的广泛收集；
- 管理指南的存储、更新及发布；
- 识别不同部门对证据的需求并分别为其提供证据服务；
- 协调患者信息服务。

Some of these tasks require the support of colleagues who manage IT. The type of work required of a knowledge manager in support of the Chief Knowledge Officer is new. It could be funded by increasing the level of investment in library services. Although there is a strong case for such increased investment, even in times of economic constraint, an alternative would be to fund librarian support for the Chief Knowledge Officer by changing the balance of tasks a librarian undertakes, for instance, changing the amount of time spent managing the library, e.g. reducing opening hours by 50%. This strategy would provide an opportunity to support the Chief Knowledge Officer and create increased value from the knowledge and skills of librarians.

■ Questions for reflection or for use in teaching or network building

If using these questions in network building or teaching, put one of the questions to the group and ask them to work in pairs to reflect on the question for three miutes; try to get people who do not know one another to work together. When taking feedback. let each pair make only one point. In the interests of equity, start with the pair on the left-hand side of the room for responses to the first question, then go to the pair on the right-hand side of the room for responses to the second question

- If you were given the responsibility of being Chief Knowledge Offcer and the necessary authority, what would be your first three actions?
- How could better use be made of the Internet as a means of managing knowledge for a population?
- If a librarian were seconded to your team or department for one day a week, what would you like them to tackle first?

References

(1) Pang, T. et al.(2006) A 15th Grand Challenge for Global Public Health. Lancet, 367: 284-286.
(2) Castells, M.(2009) The Network Society. Blackwell.
(3) Nonaka, I.(1991) The Knowledge-Creating Company. USA: Published in Harvard Business Review 1991: 14-15.
(4) Harvard Business Review on Knowledge Management(1987) Harvard Business School Press.(p.49)
(5) Grossmann, C., Goolsby, A., Olsen L. A. and McGinnis, J. M.(2007) The Learning Health Systems Series. Roundtable on Value & Science-Drive Health Care. Engineering A Learning Healthcare System. A Look at the Future. The National Academies Press.

其中的部分工作需要从事信息技术管理同事的支持。为首席知识官提供支持的知识管理者的工作类型是全新的。可以增加对图书馆服务的投资。虽然有强有力的证据表明即使是在经济拮据的时期也应当增加投资，但是还有另一种方式能够实现图书管理员对首席知识官的支持，即通过平衡图书管理员所从事的工作任务，例如，改变管理图书馆的时长，如减少图书馆50%的开放时间。这一策略可提供支持首席知识官的机会，并从图书管理员的知识和技能中创造更大的价值。

■ 互动思考题

如果在工作网络建设或教学中使用以下问题，可以将其中一个问题交给小组，让他们两人一组，思考3分钟，并尽量让彼此不认识的人一起工作。要求每组只能提出一个观点作为反馈。为了公平起见，让房间左侧的一组开始回答第1个问题，然后让房间右侧的一组开始回答第2个问题。

- 如果赋予您首席知识官的职责和必要权限，那么您的前3项行动是什么？
- 互联网作为人群知识管理的手段，如何能被更好地利用？
- 如果一个图书管理员被调派到你的团队或部门每周工作一天，你首先会让他们处理什么？

────────────────────── 参 考 文 献 ─

（6）Institute of Medicine of the National Academies（2008）Learning Healthcare System Concepts v. 2008. The Roundtable on Evidence-Based Medicine, Institute of Medicine. Annual Report（p.5）.

（7）Straus, S.E., Richardson, W.S., Glasziou, P. and Haynes, R.B.（2000）Evidence-Based Medicine. How to practice and teach EBM.（3rd Edition）Elsevier Churchill Livingstone（p.1）.

（8）Shortell, S.M. et al（2007）Improving patient care by linking evidence-based medicine and evidence-based management. JAMA, 298：673-676.

（9）Rothwell, P.M.（2007）Treating Individuals：from randomised trials to personalised medicine. Elsevier.

（10）Gigerenzer, G.（2010）Collective Statistical Illiteracy. Arch. Int. Med. 170：468.

（11）Vincent, C.（2006）Patient Safety. Churchill Livingstone（p.202）.

（12）Brook, R.H.（2010）The End of the Quality Improvement Movement. JAMA, 304：1831-1832.

（13）Friedman, M.（2005）Trying Hard is not Good Enough：how to produce measurable improvements for both customers and communities. Trafford.

（14）Moore, M.H.（1995）Creating Public Value：Strategic Management in Government. Harvard University Press.

（15）Manson N.C. and O'Neill O.（2002）Rethinking Informed Consent in Bioethics. Cambridge University Press（p.178）.

（16）Gray, J.A.M.（1998）Where is the Chief Knowledge Officer?Brit. Med.J. 317：832-833.

（17）Lyons, R.F.（2010）Using evidence：Advances and debates in bridging health research and action. Atlantic Health Promotion Research Centre.（p.12）.

（18）Gray, J.A.M.（2008）Evidence-Based Healthcare and Public Health. Elsevier.

（19）British Standards Institution（BSI）（2001）Guide to Good Practice in Knowledge Management.

（20）United Nations General Assembly（2010）Resolution adopted by the General Assembly. 64/292. The human right to water and sanitation. A/RES/64/292. 3 August 2010. Sixty-fourth session. Agenda item 48.

http：//www.un.org/ga/search/view_doc.asp?symbol＝A/RES/64/292 http：//www.un.org/waterforlifedecade/human_right_to_water.shtml

Chapter 11
CREATING AND SUSTAINING THE RIGHT CULTURE

第十一章
创建和保持正确的文化

This chapter will:

- Define what is meant by culture and subculture;
- Explain the relationship of culture to systems and structure;
- Discuss the relationship between leadership and culture;
- Describe the steps that can be taken to create an appropriate culture for the 21st century.

By the end of this chapter, you will have developed an understanding of:

- How to appraise an organisation of culture;
- The part that language plays in shaping and changing culture;
- How to assess the culture of an organisation.

Culture is one of the key components of a health service (Figure 11.1), although the paramount importance of culture in a healthcare setting has been recognised only in the last 10 years. After decades in which those who manage healthcare have been preoccupied with structure and financial regulation and, more recently, quality and safety systems, there is a need to focus explicitly on the culture of a healthcare organisation. In part, this awareness of the importance of culture resulted from the publicity about the banking scandals in 2012. In part, the revolutions in healthcare quality and safety have both led to an appreciation of the role of culture in healthcare organisations.

The quality revolution was adopted from its origins in industry, in particular from Japanese industry. The importance of managing culture, however, increased dramatically after it became obvious that there was nothing particularly 'Japanese' about the 'right' culture for continuous quality improvement (although certain aspects of Japanese life make it easier for this type of culture to develop in that country's industrial sector). The safety revolution also started in industry, specifically the aviation industry, although healthcare can be credited for recognising the importance of a safety culture as well as safety systems and of training staff to reduce preventable harm.

本章节涉及的内容：

● 定义文化和亚文化；

● 解释文化与体系和结构的关系；

● 讨论领导力与文化的关系；

● 描述可以采取哪些步骤来创建适合21世纪的文化。

在本章末，读者将会深入理解：

● 如何评价一个文化组织；

● 语言在塑造和改变文化中所起的作用；

● 如何评估一个组织的文化。

　　文化是医疗卫生服务的关键组成部分之一（图11.1），尽管人们在过去10年间才认识到文化是一个医疗卫生机构的命脉。过去的几十年间，医疗服务的管理者们一直忙于卫生体系的结构和财政规制，近些年又开始关注该体系的质量和安全问题。现在，确有必要聚焦于阐明一个医疗服务机构的文化内涵。从一定程度来说，人们对文化重要性的认识源于2012年银行业丑闻的曝光。在某种程度上，医疗服务质量和安全方面的变革都促使人们重视文化在医疗服务机构中的作用。

　　质量革命起源于工业，特别是日本工业。然而，在人们逐渐明显地意识到致力于持续改进质量的"正确"文化并无"日本"特性（尽管日本生活的某些方面使这种文化更易于在本国工业部门延展）后，管理文化的重要性则更加不言而喻。安全革命也始于工业，特别是航空业，尽管在认识到安全文化、安全系统以及培训员工以减少可预防伤害的重要性方面，可以归功于医疗服务行业。

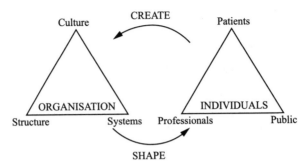

Figure 11.1 The key components of a health service

■ The meaning of 'culture'

There are almost as many meanings of the word 'culture' as there are of the term 'leadership'. When multiple meanings of a concept coexist, it is helpful to take as a reference point a definition that is widely accepted. The definition of culture probably the most highly respected and defensible is by Edgar Schein (1).

The culture of a group can now be defined as a pattern of shared basic assumptions that was learned by a group as it solved its problems of external adaptation and internal integration, that has worked well enough to be considered valid and, therefore, to be taught to new members as the correct way to perceive, think, and feel in relation to those problems. (1)

Another example of a definition for the term 'culture' is used is that by a British team, which highlights that culture influences not only decision-making in an organisation but also the way in which people behave:

...assumptions, values and patterns of behaviour within an organization are often termed its 'organizational culture'. (2)

It is important to be aware of and recognise the presence of any subcultures within the culture of a health service. The existence of subcultures is determined by three principal influences.

1. The power of national or international cultures relating to a particular specialty: in every country, the culture of a cardiothoracic service is different from that of a paediatric service, and both differ from the culture of a mental health service.

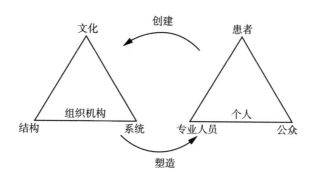

图11.1 卫生服务的关键组成部分

■"文化"的含义

"文化"一词的含义几乎和"领导力"一词的含义一样多。当一个概念有多种含义并存时，以一个被广泛接受的定义作为参考点是有助于对其的理解。埃德加·沙因对文化的定义大概是最受推崇和最站得住脚[1]。

一个群体的文化现在可以被定义为一种共享基本设想的模式，这种模式由该群体在解决外部适应和内部整合问题时习得，运作良好，足以被认为是有效的。因此，将它教导给新成员，作为看待、思考和感受这些问题的正确方式。[1]

另一个关于"文化"定义的例子来自一个英国团队，它强调文化不仅影响一个组织机构的决策，而且也影响人们的行为方式：

……组织内的设想、价值观和行为模式通常被称为"组织文化"。[2]

还有重要的一点是，要意识到并认同在一个医疗卫生服务的文化内存在着各种亚文化。这些亚文化的存在受到了以下3个主要因素的影响。

1. 与特定专业相关的国家或国际文化的力量：在每个国家，心胸外科服务的文化都不同于儿科服务的文化，而且两者都不同于心理健康服务的文化。

2. The nature of the prevailing leadership, for instance, the culture of a particular cardiothoracic or paediatric service may differ greatly from that of another within the same health service — walking from one ward to another can be like going from France to Italy.

3. The development of countercultures in opposition to the culture created by the official leadership of an organisation. There are two main types of counterculture: formal and informal. The Board of a hospital may regard the trade union as a counterculture, but it has a formal standing. An informal counterculture in a hospital might be one of heavy drinking, or there may a racist subculture.

If multiple meanings of a term do co-exist, it is advisable to take a few minutes at the beginning of any meeting at which culture is discussed to clarify the meaning to be used. Although Edgar Schein's definition can be offered at the outset, it is better to ask participants to work in pairs for two minutes to identify what they believe to be the key points in the definition of culture. For the majority of such discussions, a sufficient number of 'hooks' will be identified for the Schein definition to be adopted by the group. When initiating the discussion, by way of introduction, it can be helpful:

- *to use the commonsense and commonplace definition of culture as 'the way things are done around here'*;
- *to encourage people to reflect on different wards, hospitals or health centres in order to identify elements of culture that may be obvious when we walk into those environments.*

■ Assessing culture

In *Language, Truth and Logic*, A.J. Ayer emphasised that although words could be used to explain meaning, another approach was through measurement (3). Ayer said that:

...the meaning of a proposition is determined by the observations one would make to confirm or refute the truth of that proposition.

2. 占主导地位领导力的性质，例如，某特定团队的胸外科服务或儿科服务的文化，可能与在同一系统中的另外服务团队的文化大不相同——从一个病房走到另一个病房，简直像从法国到了意大利。

3. 与组织内官方领导者所创立文化相对立的反主流文化的发展状况。反主流文化主要有两种类型：正式的和非正式的。医院董事会可能把工会视为一种反主流文化，但工会具有正式的地位。在某医院里，非正式的反主流文化之一可能是酗酒，或是存在某种种族主义亚文化。

如果一个术语同时存在多种含义，建议在任何讨论文化的会议开始时花几分钟来阐明要使用的术语的含义。虽然可以在会议开始时就给出埃德加·沙因对文化的定义，但最好邀请与会者两人一组，花两分钟的时间确定他们所认为的文化定义中的关键点。大多数此类讨论可以发现足够数量的与定义相关联的"结合点"，以供该群体采纳埃德加·沙因的定义。当开始讨论时，通过介绍的方式，做到以下两点可能会有所帮助：

● 使用常识和通俗的文化定义即"在这里，就是如此行事的"（入乡随俗的意思）；

● 鼓励人们对不同的病房、医院或健康中心进行反思，以识别哪些文化元素是走进这些环境时就扑面而来、使我们能明显感受到的。

■ 评估文化

艾耶尔在《语言，真理和逻辑》一书中强调，虽然可以用词语对含义进行解释，不过也可以使用测量的方法[3]。艾耶尔说：

……一个命题的意义是由为了证实或反驳该命题的真实性而进行的观察所决定的。

Propositions such as 'We value diversity' or 'We have a culture of patient-centred care' are commonplace, but how can their truth be determined? There are three main approaches to appraising an organisation's culture.

1. Reading the documents produced and other platforms, e.g. the prospectus or brochure, leaflets for patients, the annual report and the website: such documents reflect the expressed culture, explicitly, through what is articulated, and implicitly for what is absent or lacks emphasis — documents and other platforms, however, are not the only source of information about a culture, and they are probably the least reliable even though a great deal of thought has gone into their production;

2. Observing what Edgar Schein called 'the artefacts of an organisation' (see Box 11.1), which tend to be related to the physical environment: this approach is more likely to produce reliable results than document analysis because less thought has gone into managing the impression organisational artefacts will make on an outsider; however, the physical environment of a service is a fairly coarse measure of culture, and it may be more fruitful to observe and assess staff behaviour not only towards patients but also towards one another;

3. Listening to people who work in or use an organisation: listening is a way of collecting knowledge derived from experience, which can be a rich source of information for culture change. Anthropologists seek out people they call 'informants', namely, knowledgeable insiders who are willing to be interviewed; however, an informant's account may be biased, and the reasons for bias may not be revealed to the enquirer. Furthermore, the process of listening and observing can change how people behave or what they say, depending on the status of the enquirer and the informant's perception of the purpose of the enquiry.

Box 11.1 Examples of artefacts in a health service organisation

- Are the patient toilets as clean as the staff toilets?
- Is the waiting room decorated in the same way as the Board Room?
- Does the Chief Executive have a designated car-park space close to the front door of the hospital?

诸如"我们重视多元性"或"我们有以患者为中心的医疗文化"这样的主张是司空见惯的，但如何确定他们的真实性呢？评估一个组织机构的文化主要有以下3种方法：

1. 查阅机构制作的文件和其他平台，例如说明书或手册、为患者提供的印刷品、年度报告和网站，因为这些文件通过明确内容反映了其表达的文化，并含蓄地反映了缺少或未强调的内容。不过，文件和其他平台提供的内容并不是关于一种文化的唯一信息来源，它们可能是最不可靠的，尽管在它们的制作过程中花费了大量的心思。

2. 观察埃德加·沙因所称的"一个组织机构的人工建制（artefact）"[①]（专栏11.1），其往往与物质（硬件）环境有关：这种方法比文档分析更有可能产生可靠的结果，因为很少有人会考虑如何管理组织机构的人工制品给外人留下的印象。然而，一个服务机构的外部（硬件）环境是一种对文化相当粗糙的衡量，而观察和评估员工对患者和对同事之间的行为，则可能更有收获。

3. 倾听在组织中工作或利用该组织的人员：倾听是从经验中收集知识的一种方式，可以成为文化变革的丰富信息来源。人类学家寻找他们称之为"线人"的人，即愿意接受采访的有见识的内部人士。然而，线人的叙述可能有偏倚，且可能不会向调查者透露偏倚的原因。此外，倾听和观察的过程可能会改变人们的行为或他们所说的话，这取决于调查者的状态和线人对调查目的的看法。

专栏11.1　卫生服务机构的人工建制示例

- 患者的厕所和员工的厕所一样干净吗？
- 候诊室的装修方式和董事会会议室一样吗？
- 行政长官是否在医院前门附近设有指定停车位？

[①] 译者注：组织的人工建制（artefact）是指对组织的所有利益相关者都有意义的材料、建筑、符号、名称、图像、标识、流行语。

Although it is becoming common for Chief Executives in the business sector to visit frontline operations unrecognised, this method of observing organisational culture is more difficult in the health service because in a hospital a Chief Executive is more likely to be recognised by frontline staff.

■ Mutual learning

It is difficult to learn about the culture in which one works because any culture institutionalises those who work within it. One way to circumvent this difficulty is to take a mutual learning approach.

Apply the 'buddy' system and work with someone in another organization so that each person can act as the key informant about the culture of the other's organisation. A simple template that can be used for reporting these findings (see Display 11. 1); it can also be used within your own organisation. Without reflecting on culture change, improvement is not possible.

■ Culture and leadership

Culture and leadership are inter-related:

When we examine culture and leadership closely, we see that they are two sides of the same coin; neither can really be understood by itself. If one wishes to distinguish leadership from management or administration, one can argue that leadership creates and changes cultures, while management and administration act within a culture. (4)

This principle is very important to successful organisations like Toyota because:

An organization's culture defines what goes on in its workplace. Loosely defined, culture is the soft, imprecise, fuzzy stuff of everyday life. Within any company, it is what people think and believe and what drives daily priorities. Leadership and a company's culture are inextricably intertwined. (5)

尽管商业部门的首席执行官们在未被认出来的情况下访问前线运营部门已变得司空见惯，但这种观察组织文化的方法在医疗服务部门较为困难，因为在医院，首席执行官更容易被一线员工认出来。

■ 相互学习

要了解某一个人工作的文化是很困难的，因为任何一种文化都将在其中工作的人"体制化"了。规避这一困难的一种方法是采取相互学习的方式。应用"同伴"系统，与另一个组织中的某个人合作，这样每个人都可以充当对方组织文化的"线人"。可使用一个简单的模板来报告这些发现（场景11.1），该模板也可在您本人所在的组织内使用。若缺乏对文化变革的反思，则无法进步。

■ 文化和领导力

文化和领导力是有内在关联的。

当我们仔细审视文化和领导力时，我们会发现它们是一枚硬币的两面，两者凭其自身并不能被真正理解。如果有人想将领导力与管理或行政区分开来，那可以说，领导力创造和改变着文化，而行政管理则是在文化中发挥作用。[4]

此原理对丰田公司这类成功的企业而言非常重要。因为：

一个组织的文化界定了其工作场所该如何运营。从广义上讲，文化指的是每天日常生活中那些软性的、难以精确表达和模糊的内容。在任何一家公司里，文化是人们所想所信以及日常重点工作的驱动力。领导力与企业文化是密不可分的。[5]

Display 11.1

Method of appraisal	Observations
Reading ● What struck me about the culture of this organisation from reading its documents? ● What impressed me favourably? ● What was missing? ● What dismayed me?	
Looking ● From my observations, were there any signals about the way in which this organisation regards its staff and its patients?	
Listening When speaking with people: ● What did I learn about the culture of the organisation? ● Did what I hear differ from what I read in the documents?	

Despite the multiple meaning, of the words 'culture' and 'leadership', there is a common thread among them: many of the definitions emphasise that leaders shape culture whereas managers work within it. For the clinician with an interest in population medicine, being a leader and therefore shaping culture is part of the job.

■ Creating a new culture

Clinicians in leadership positions have a responsibility for changing all aspects of culture. The shift in healthcare provision from a paradigm in which the concern is with those patients in contact with a service to one in which the concern is for the population served requires a considerable cultural change. A culture with the whole population as its concern exhibits the characteristics shown in Box 11.2.

场景11.1

评价方法	观察结果
查阅 ● 通过查阅其管理制度相关文件，这个组织的文化给我留下了哪些深刻印象？ ● 哪些方面给我留下良好的印象？ ● 哪些方面是缺失的？ ● 哪些方面让我感到沮丧？	
观察 ● 根据我在现场的观察，是否捕获到任何有关该组织对待其员工和患者的方式的重要信息？	
倾听 当与该组织机构的员工交谈时： ● 关于这个组织的文化我了解到了什么？ ● 我听到的与我从文件中读到的各种内容有区别吗？	

尽管"文化"和"领导力"这两个词有多种含义，但它们之间有一条共同的主线：许多定义都强调领导者塑造文化，而管理者在文化中则扮演执行的角色。对于热衷于群医学的临床医生而言，作为领导者并因此塑造文化，则是其工作的一部分。

■创立新文化

处于领导岗位的临床医生有责任改变文化的各个方面。在医疗供给方面，从关注就诊患者转向关注所有人群这一范式的转变，需要进行重大的文化变革。如专栏11.2所示，"关注整个人群"的文化具有如下特征。

Box 11.2 Characteristics of a healthcare culture concerned with the population served

- In documents describing the service, there are frequent references to the population served, and not only reports about the quality of care delivered to the proportion of the population in contact with the service but also about the whole population in need, the level of unmet need, and degree of variation in referral rates to the hospital service according to referring practice and socio-economic group of patient.
- Maps are the artefacts that indicate whether a service is concerned with the population. Although maps are rarely visible in hospitals, the service providing care for a population will have numerous maps on display, which provide a key source of information for a population-based health service: for example, maps showing isochrones of the time taken to travel to the hospital from different housing estates in the locality, subpopulations in which there is a high incidence of disease or from which there is a high referral rate. The identification of variation often reveals cultural differences.

This shift in paradigm, however, is one change among several that need to take place if the culture of healthcare organisations is to be transformed from that which was appropriate for the 20th century to that which is appropriate for the 21st century. The various shifts in health service culture that need to take place are summarised in Figure 11.2.

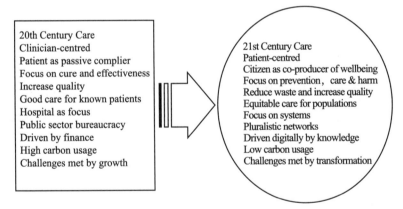

Figure 11.2 The transformation in 20th century healthcare culture to meet the needs of the 21st century

■ Creating a culture of respect

It is common for clinicians in specialist services to speak with disrespect of clinicians in generalist service, often without experience of having worked in general practice:

专栏 11.2 与所服务人群有关的医疗卫生文化特征

- 在描述医疗卫生服务的文件中，经常会引用到"所服务人群"的信息；内容不仅涉及直接受益人群（如患者，仅占此人群的一部分）所获得的卫生服务的质量，也涉及那些有需要的全体人群，人群未满足的医疗卫生需求，以及医院转诊率根据转诊实践和社会经济群体而变化的程度。
- 从绘制的各类路径图中，可以看出该服务是否真正关注到了应该涉及的人群。尽管在医院里很少能看到此类路径图，但为人群提供的医疗卫生服务中，此类路径图却处处可见且提供了重要的信息。例如，可绘制当地从不同住宅区到医院所花时间的等时线地图，发病率高或转诊率高的亚人群所在位置。这些差异的识别往往可以揭示出文化的不同。

然而，如果要将医疗卫生机构的文化从适合20世纪转变为适合于21世纪，范式的转变仅是诸多需要进行的变革之一。图11.2总结了卫生服务文化中需要发生的几类变革。

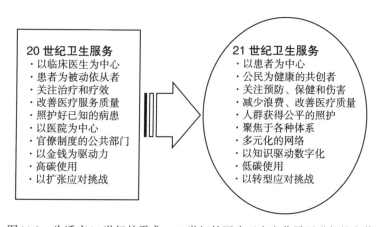

图 11.2 为适应21世纪的需求，20世纪的医疗卫生文化需要进行的变革

■ 创建一种"尊重"的文化

一个常见的状况是，专科医生虽然没有在全科领域的工作经验，却经常会对从事全科医生出言不逊。

'I can't think why we don't see more stroke patients. It is a dead easy diagnosis to make — a typical headache in someone of middle age.'

This specialist, however, has failed to understand an important epidemiological distinction between the sensitivity of a test and its positive predictive value. To the specialist neurosurgeon, the diagnosis is easy because 90% of people who have a stroke of a certain type report this history; however, if general practitioners referred every middle-aged person with atypical headache, the specialist service would be flooded because the positive predictive value of that collection of symptoms is much lower in general practice.

There is a need to move towards a culture in which clinicians in specialist services speak with respect of clinicians in the generalist service because in population medicine all clinicians are of equal standing although they may perform different jobs.

■ The influence of leadership

Any leader influences culture through what they say and, importantly, through the way in which they behave. For clinicians leading a service concerned with the population served, it is essential to control:

- *the editorial content of any documents produced;*
- *the appearance of buildings relevant to the health service and the environment in which care is provided.*

When embarking upon culture change, these aspects of the service convey messages about the organisation's culture, not only to the population served but also to the wider general public.

It is important to be explicit about culture. Ten years ago it would have been rare to discuss the culture of an organisation, whereas now it is common and should be universal. Although the leaders of an organisation must be aware of their behaviour, but they also need to think more about the language they use because language is the dominant determinant in the culture of an organisation. It is also the main way in which culture is conveyed to people who come into contact with the organisation or people who join it. Although the concept of an organisation's 'culture' can sometimes seem nebulous, there are discrete explicit steps that

"我不明白为什么我们没有看到更多的脑卒中患者。这是一个非常容易做出的诊断——中年人的非典型头痛。"

然而这位专科医生未能理解检查的灵敏度与阳性预测值之间重要的流行病学区别。对于神经外科专科医生来说，做出诊断很容易，因为90%患有某种类型的脑卒中的患者有过这种症状；然而，在全科医学门诊中这些症状的阳性预测值要低得多，如果全科医生将每个患有非典型头痛的中年人转诊，那么患者将大量地涌入专科服务。

文化建设应当朝着这么一个方向发展：从事专科的临床医生尊重从事全科的医生。因为在群医学中，所有临床医生虽然可能从事着不同的工作，但他们的地位一律平等。

■ 领导者的影响

任何一名领导者都会通过其言论——更为重要的是通过其行为方式——来影响所在组织机构的文化。对于为人群提供医疗服务的临床医生而言，有必要对以下方面进行管控：

- 组织机构编制的任何文件的内容；
- 与医疗服务相关的建筑物外观以及提供医疗卫生服务的环境。

当进行文化变革时，这些服务内容不仅向所服务的人群，也向广大民众传递了与机构文化相关的信息。

精准阐明文化内容十分重要。如果说十年前探讨组织文化还十分罕见，那么现在这已变得常见，而且还应推广普及。尽管一个组织的领导者们不仅必须意识到其行为对机构文化的影响，他们也需更多地考虑所使用的语言，因为语言是组织文化中的主要决定因素。这也是将文化传达给外部接触者或内部人员的主要方式。虽然一个组织的"文化"概念有时看起来模糊不清，

can be taken to influence culture by shaping the language used and the concepts that prevail.

Although the behaviour of the leadership is important in creating a new culture, or in shaping an existing culture, it is necessary to complement behaviour at a leadership level with measures to ensure that people are cognisant of the culture change and act accordingly.

■ The role of language

When creating a new culture, it is important to examine the language used in an organisation. It is particularly helpful to identify:

- *terms that should not be used, such as 'bed blocker';*
- *terms that need to be used consistently because they are important to the development of a common set of principles and assumptions, e.g. 'quality' and 'efficiency'. If a term is in common use, it is likely that it has multiple meanings, even within a small management team.*

Questions that can be used to identify whether there is a need to create a common language and a set of shared concepts for an organization are shown in Box 11.3.

Box 11.3 Questions to ascertain whether a common language is needed in an organisation

- If all the key people in the organisation were asked to write down what they meant by patient-centred care, how consistent would the answers be?
- If the leadership team were asked to write down what they meant by the term 'value' and how the meaning differed from that of 'quality', what would they write?
- If all the lead clinicians were asked to describe what they understood by the terms 'inappropriate' care and 'optimal use of resources', how diverse would the ansevers be?

Language is also shaped by the concepts expressed in books and articles. In addition to a conventional journal club, it would be helpful to establish a 21st Century Book Club. In this type of book club, it is not necessary for everyone to have read the book; instead, the person who has read a book which they regard as important, or has been important to them, describes the key messages as a basis

但仍可采用具体精准的步骤——包括塑造所用语言和各种主流理念——来影响文化。

尽管在创造新文化或打造现有文化方面，领导者的行为很重要，但仍有必要在高级管理层的文化方面采取额外措施，以确保所有人都认识到文化的变化并按其行事。

■ 语言的作用

当建立一种新的文化时，很重要的一点是要审视组织中使用的语言，这特别有助于辨认：

- 不应该使用的术语，如"病房钉子户"；
- 需要持续使用的术语，因为它们对于制定一套通用的原则和假设来说很重要，例如"质量"和"效率"。如果一个术语很常用，那么它很可能有多种含义，即使在一个小的管理团队中也是如此。

专栏11.3展示了一些问题，用来确定是否需要为组织创建一种通用语言和一组共享概念。

专栏11.3　用以确定组织中是否需要一种通用语言的问题

- 如果要求组织中的所有关键人员写下他们所说的以患者为中心的医疗照护的含义，答案的一致性如何？
- 如果要求领导团队写下他们对"价值"一词的理解，以及这个词与"质量"的含义有何不同，他们会写什么？
- 如果要求所有的主任医师阐述他们对"不适当的医疗照护"和"最优的资源利用"两个术语的理解，会有多少种答案？

语言也是受到书籍和文章中表达的概念的影响而形成的。除了一个常规的期刊俱乐部，成立一个21世纪的读书俱乐部也很有帮助。在这种读书俱乐部中，不一定每个人都已经读过某本书；而是，某人读过一本大家认为很重

for discussion and reflection.

'Culture eats strategy for breakfast' is the traditional management proverb. More than that, it eats structural reorganisation for lunch, dinner and afternoon tea!

■ Questions for reflection or for use in teaching or network building

If using these questions in network building or teaching, put one of the questions to the group and ask them to work in pairs to reflect on the question for three minutes; try to get people who do not know one another to work together. When taking feedback, let each pair make only one point. In the interests of equity, start with the pair on the left-hand side of the room for responses to the first question, then go to the pair on the right-hand side of the room for responses to the second question.

- How well does your website reflect your official culture?
- If a colleague from another service or hospital went to visit your facility, which aspects of culture would be viewed favourably and which would be viewed unfavourably for an organisation that claims 'to put patients first' ?
- What book or individual has had the greatest influence on your work in healthcare, and why?

References

(1) Schein, E.H. (2004) Organizational Culture and Leadership. John Wiley & Sons Inc. (p.17).

(2) Mannion, R., Davies, H.T.O., Marshall, M.N. (2005) Cultures for Performance in Health Care. Open University Press. (p.1).

(3) Ayer, A.J. (1935) Language, Truth and Logic. Penguin.

要的或者大家认为很重要的书，之后可以描述某些关键的信息来作为讨论和反思的基础，对大家很重要。

"文化能把战略当早餐吃"，这是一句经典的管理学谚语。不止如此，文化还会把结构重组当午饭、晚饭甚至下午茶。

■ 互动思考题

如果在工作网络建设或教学中使用以下问题，可以将其中一个问题交给小组，让他们两人一组，思考3分钟，并尽量让彼此不认识的人一起工作。要求每组只能提出一个观点作为反馈。为了公平起见，让房间左侧的一组开始回答第1个问题，然后让房间右侧的一组开始回答第2个问题。

- 您的网站多大程度上反映了官方文化？
- 如果来自其他服务部门或医院的同事来参观您的机构，对于一个声称"将患者放在首位"的组织来说，哪些方面的文化会被认为是有利的，哪些会被认为是不利的？
- 哪本书或哪个人对您的医疗工作产生的影响最大？为什么？

───────────────── 参 考 文 献 ─

（4）Schein, E.H.（2004）Organizational Culture and Leadership. John Wiley & Sons Inc.（pp.10-11）.

（5）Morgan, J.M. and Liker, J.K.（2006）The Toyota Product Development System. Integrating people, process, and technology. Productivity Press, New York, pp.217, 218.